50 Studies Every Neurologist Should Know

50 STUDIES EVERY DOCTOR SHOULD KNOW

Published and Forthcoming Books in the *50 Studies Every Doctor Should Know* Series

50 Studies Every Doctor Should Know: The Key Studies that Form the Foundation of Evidence Based Medicine, Revised Edition
Michael E. Hochman

50 Studies Every Internist Should Know
Kristopher Swiger, Joshua R. Thomas, Michael E. Hochman, and Steven D. Hochman

50 Studies Every Neurologist Should Know
David Y. Hwang and David M. Greer

50 Studies Every Surgeon Should Know
SreyRam Kuy and Rachel J. Kwon

50 Studies Every Pediatrician Should Know
Ashaunta Anderson, Nina L. Shapiro, Stephen C. Aronoff, Jeremiah Davis, and Michael Levy

50 Imaging Studies Every Doctor Should Know
Christoph Lee

50 Studies Every Anesthesiologist Should Know
Anita Gupta

50 Studies Every Intensivist Should Know
Edward Bittner

50 Studies Every Psychiatrist Should Know
Vinod Srihari, Ish Bhalla, and Rajesh Tampi

50 Studies Every Neurologist Should Know

EDITED BY

David Y. Hwang, MD

Assistant Professor of Neurology
Division of Neurocritical Care and Emergency Neurology
Yale School of Medicine
New Haven, Connecticut

David M. Greer, MD, MA

Zimmerman and Spinelli Professor and Vice Chairman of Neurology
Yale School of Medicine
New Haven, Connecticut

SERIES EDITOR:

Michael E. Hochman, MD, MPH

Assistant Professor of Clinical Medicine
Keck School of Medicine
University of Southern California
Los Angeles, California

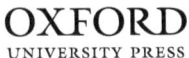

OXFORD
UNIVERSITY PRESS

Oxford University Press is a department of the University of Oxford. It furthers the University's objective of excellence in research, scholarship, and education by publishing worldwide. Oxford is a registered trade mark of Oxford University Press in the UK and certain other countries.

Published in the United States of America by Oxford University Press
198 Madison Avenue, New York, NY 10016, United States of America.

© Oxford University Press 2016

First Edition published in 2016

All rights reserved. No part of this publication may be reproduced, stored in a retrieval system, or transmitted, in any form or by any means, without the prior permission in writing of Oxford University Press, or as expressly permitted by law, by license, or under terms agreed with the appropriate reproduction rights organization. Inquiries concerning reproduction outside the scope of the above should be sent to the Rights Department, Oxford University Press, at the address above.

You must not circulate this work in any other form
and you must impose this same condition on any acquirer.

Library of Congress Cataloging-in-Publication Data
50 studies every neurologist should know / edited by David Y. Hwang, David M. Greer.
 p. ; cm. — (50 studies every doctor should know)
Fifty studies every neurologist should know
Includes bibliographical references.
ISBN 978–0–19–937752–7 (alk. paper)
I. Hwang, David Y., editor. II. Greer, David M., 1966– , editor. III. Title: Fifty studies every neurologist should know. IV. Series: 50 studies every doctor should know (Series)
 [DNLM: 1. Nervous System Diseases—drug therapy. 2. Clinical Medicine—methods. 3. Clinical Trials as Topic. WL 140]
RC337
616.8′0427—dc23
2015035661

This material is not intended to be, and should not be considered, a substitute for medical or other professional advice. Treatment for the conditions described in this material is highly dependent on the individual circumstances. And, while this material is designed to offer accurate information with respect to the subject matter covered and to be current as of the time it was written, research and knowledge about medical and health issues is constantly evolving and dose schedules for medications are being revised continually, with new side effects recognized and accounted for regularly. Readers must therefore always check the product information and clinical procedures with the most up-to-date published product information and data sheets provided by the manufacturers and the most recent codes of conduct and safety regulation. The publisher and the authors make no representations or warranties to readers, express or implied, as to the accuracy or completeness of this material. Without limiting the foregoing, the publisher and the authors make no representations or warranties as to the accuracy or efficacy of the drug dosages mentioned in the material. The authors and the publisher do not accept, and expressly disclaim, any responsibility for any liability, loss, or risk that may be claimed or incurred as a consequence of the use and/or application of any of the contents of this material.

CONTENTS

Preface xi
Acknowledgments xiii
Contributors xix

SECTION 1 Behavioral Neurology

1. Cholinesterase Inhibitors for Alzheimer's Disease   3
   Ashish L. Ranpura

2. Memantine for Alzheimer's Disease   11
   Joshua Lovinger

SECTION 2 Epilepsy

3. Lorazepam for Generalized Status Epilepticus   21
   Pue Farooque

4. Lamotrigine for Partial Epilepsy: Arm A of the SANAD Trial   27
   Amy Chan

5. Valproate for Generalized and Unclassifiable Epilepsy: Arm B of the SANAD Trial   33
   Shivani Ghoshal

SECTION 3 Headache

6. Sumatriptan for Acute Migraine   41
   Allison Arch

SECTION 4 Neuroinfectious Disease

7. Steroids for Bell's Palsy   49
   Benjamin N. Blond

8. Steroids for Acute Bacterial Meningitis   55
   Robert J. Claycomb

SECTION 5 Movement Disorders

9. Levodopa for Parkinson's Disease   63
   Sarah E. Buckingham

10. Deep-Brain Stimulation for Parkinson's Disease   71
    Sarah E. Buckingham

SECTION 6 Multiple Sclerosis

11. Oral vs. IV Steroids for Acute Relapses of Multiple Sclerosis   81
    Joshua Lovinger

12. Interferon Beta-1a for a First Demyelinating Event:
    The CHAMPS Trial   87
    Sarah A. Mulukutla

13. Glatiramer Acetate for Clinically Isolated Syndrome:
    The PreCISe Trial   93
    Sarah A. Mulukutla

14. Natalizumab for Relapsing Multiple Sclerosis:
    The SENTINEL Trial   99
    Robert J. Claycomb

15. Fingolimod for Relapsing Multiple Sclerosis:
    The TRANSFORMS Trial   105
    Mary A. Bailey

16. Oral BG-12 for Relapsing-Remitting Multiple Sclerosis,
    Part I: The DEFINE Trial   111
    Mary A. Bailey

17. Oral BG-12 for Relapsing-Remitting Multiple Sclerosis,
    Part II: The CONFIRM Trial   115
    Mary A. Bailey

SECTION 7 Neurocritical Care

18. Therapeutic Hypothermia for Cardiac Arrest,
    Part I: The HACA Trial   123
    Teddy S. Youn

19. Therapeutic Hypothermia for Cardiac Arrest,
    Part II: The Australian Trial   129
    Teddy S. Youn

20. Decompressive Craniectomy for Diffuse Traumatic Brain
    Injury: The DECRA Trial   135
    Shivani Ghoshal

21. Nimodipine for Subarachnoid Hemorrhage   141
    Teddy S. Youn

SECTION 8 Neuromuscular Disease

22. IVIG vs. Plasma Exchange for Guillain-Barré Syndrome   151
    Irene Hwa Yang

23. IVIG versus Plasma Exchange for Myasthenia Gravis   157
    Kimberly R. Robeson

24. Riluzole for Amyotrophic Lateral Sclerosis   163
    Brian Mac Grory

SECTION 9 Neuro-Oncology

25. Radiotherapy Plus Temozolomide for Glioblastoma   171
    Amy Chan

26. Methylated *MGMT* Gene Promoter and Response
    to Temozolomide for Glioblastoma   177
    Joshua Lovinger

SECTION 10 Neuro-Ophthalmology

27. Steroids for Acute Optic Neuritis: The Optic Neuritis
    Treatment Trial   185
    Mary A. Bailey

SECTION 11 Neuro-Otology

28. The Epley Maneuver for Benign Paroxysmal Positional Vertigo   193
    Benjamin N. Blond

SECTION 12 Sleep

29. Modafinil for Narcolepsy   203
    Abeer J. Hani

30. Continuous Dopamine Agonist for Restless Legs Syndrome   209
    Ashish L. Ranpura

SECTION 13 Spine Disorders

31. Early Surgery for Sciatica   219
    Luis Kolb

32. Surgery for Lumbar Degenerative Spondylolisthesis: The SPORT Trial   225
    Ryan A. Grant

33. Steroids versus No Steroids for Acute Spinal Cord Injury: The NASCIS II Trial   233
    Sacit Bulent Omay

SECTION 14 Vascular Neurology

34. IV Thrombolysis 3 Hours after an Acute Ischemic Stroke: The NINDS Trial   241
    Hardik P. Amin

35. IV Thrombolysis 3 to 4.5 Hours after an Acute Ischemic Stroke: The ECASS III Trial   247
    Michael E. Hochman

36. Endovascular Therapy for Acute Ischemic Stroke, Part I (Intra-arterial Thrombolysis): The PROACT II Trial   253
    Allison Arch and *David Y. Hwang*

37. Endovascular Therapy for Acute Ischemic Stroke, Part II (After IV Thrombolysis): The IMS III Trial   259
    Matthew D. Kalp and *David Y. Hwang*

38. Endovascular Therapy for Acute Ischemic Stroke, Part III (Using Neuroimaging to Select Patients): The MR RESCUE Trial   265
    Matthew D. Kalp and David Y. Hwang

39. Endovascular Therapy for Acute Ischemic Stroke, Part IV (Clinical Trial Success): The MR CLEAN Trial   271
    Matthew D. Kalp and David Y. Hwang

40. Carotid Endarterectomy for Symptomatic High-Grade Carotid Stenosis: The NASCET Trial, Part I   277
    Hardik P. Amin

41. Carotid Endarterectomy for Symptomatic Moderate Carotid Stenosis: The NASCET Trial, Part II   283
    Hardik P. Amin

42. Carotid Endarterectomy for Asymptomatic Carotid Stenosis: The ACAS Trial   289
    Daniel C. Brooks

43. Early Aspirin for Acute Ischemic Stroke: The CAST Trial   295
    Mark Landreneau

44. Aspirin vs. Heparin for Acute Ischemic Stroke: The IST Trial   299
    Mark Landreneau

45. Dipyridamole and Aspirin for Secondary Stroke Prevention: The ESPS-2 Trial   305
    Robert J. Claycomb

46. High-Dose Atorvastatin after Stroke or Transient Ischemic Attack: The SPARCL Trial   311
    Brian Mac Grory

47. Adjusted-Dose Warfarin for Stroke Prevention in High-Risk Atrial Fibrillation Patients: The SPAF III Trial   317
    Daniel C. Brooks

48. Dabigatran for Stroke Prevention in Atrial Fibrillation Patients: The RE-LY Trial   323
    Robert J. Claycomb

49. Apixaban for Stroke Prevention in Atrial Fibrillation Patients: The ARISTOTLE Trial   329
    Daniel C. Brooks

50. Rivaroxaban for Stroke Prevention in Atrial Fibrillation Patients: The ROCKET AF Trial   335
    Daniel C. Brooks

Index   341

PREFACE

Much emphasis is placed on lesion localization in the clinical neurosciences—and rightfully so. Medical students worldwide spend countless hours committing the central and peripheral functional neuroanatomy found in textbooks to memory. From brainstem stroke syndromes to the circuitry of the brachial plexus, mastering the pathways of the nervous system is the classic starting point in caring for patients with neurologic illness.

Yet, even the most well-prepared new neurology resident finds out very quickly when he or she begins their first rotation that localizing a patient's lesion—while not always straightforward, even with neuroimaging—is only the beginning of patient care. In particular, there has been an explosion of clinical trials in the past 50 years in neurology that has given our field more treatments than ever before. This explosion has also made it more difficult to start as a new neurologist and attempt to build expertise in evidence-based medicine from scratch. Figuring out what to do for patients, and why to do it, is a never-ending process for all physicians, and it is particularly daunting for certain groups, such as the first-year neurology resident who is making the transition from internship, or the new senior neurology resident who is attempting to lead a team for the very first time. Even for the generalist who is beginning his or her first practice, or the seasoned academic specialist who finds himself or herself bracing for a month on the ward service, feeling confident in one's knowledge base of foundational studies in clinical neurology is no easy task.

No one book can provide what can only be acquired through years of reading and clinical experience. However, in the spirit of Oxford's *50 Studies* series, the purpose of this book is to provide an introduction to key clinical trials in neurology that have impacted practice. It is meant as a starting point, so that one may walk into rounds or a case conference and feel more confident that they have an idea of *why* we do *what* we do. By design, each chapter summarizes a trial or a group of trials in a format that is brief enough to be reasonably digested by a resident while on a busy service, yet comprehensive enough that not only the results but the generalizability of each trial is emphasized. In fact, some of the papers summarized no longer represent our standard of care, but their initial impact on practice was dramatic enough that they are still shaping the narrative about how certain diseases are treated. Our hope is that the book will fill a need for trainees (and perhaps for practicing neurologists): a manual that places treatments for neurologic diseases into context and that allows one to drink from the fire hydrant that is clinical neurology perhaps a little more easily.

The biggest issue with putting together a book such as this one is figuring out which 50 studies to include. While the selection of studies for this book were peer reviewed by a national committee of educators in neurology, the bottom line is that we picked studies that simply seem to come up on rounds frequently. Fair or not, we also emphasized subspecialties that happen to have a number of large multicenter clinical trials. One glance at the table of contents will reveal that the book is thus heavily weighted toward inpatient neurology and, in particular, vascular neurology. The fact that some subspecialties have much fewer studies represented is by no means a reflection of their importance in neurology, but rather a recognition that, for better or for worse, almost every neurologist is responsible for taking care of stroke patients because of their sheer prevalence on our services!

As an initial volume, we consider this book a work in progress—we welcome your thoughts as to the studies that have been included or excluded, and believe that if the book has future editions, opportunities to refine its contents will exist. While starting a debate over which studies are most impactful is interesting, it is our wish that this book makes the foundations of evidence-based clinical neurology a little less overwhelming to someone who is starting out. Thanks very much for picking up this book; we very much hope that you find it useful.

David Y. Hwang, MD
David M. Greer, MD, MA

ACKNOWLEDGMENTS

This book was only made possible by the collective efforts of our contributors: by and large, the residents and faculty in the Departments of Neurology and Neurosurgery at the Yale School of Medicine. Many thanks for the hours of work that they put into writing and revising the chapters of this book.

We thank Dr. Michael Hochman, the *50 Studies* series editor, and Oxford University Press for the opportunity to make this unique book a reality. We also thank the anonymous peer-review panel of neurologic educators recruited by OUP who helped us hone our list of studies and who recommended publication.

Finally, we would like to thank the following reviewers, who were kind enough to spend time reviewing the content of this book. Many of these reviewers are authors of the studies that are summarized. For those chapters for which an original study author was not available, and the subject was in a subspecialty outside of stroke and neurocritical care, we recruited additional expert faculty for assistance with content review. We are very grateful to all. Importantly, however, the views expressed in this book do not represent those of the authors and reviewers acknowledged hereafter, nor do these authors vouch for the accuracy of the information; any mistakes are our own.

David Y. Hwang, MD
David M. Greer, MD, MA

- Dr. Lawrence T. Friedhoff, senior author: A 24-week, double-blind, placebo-controlled trial of donepezil in patients with Alzheimer's disease. Donepezil Study Group. *Neurology*. 1998;50:136–145. We also appreciate Dr. Darren C. Volpe, Assistant Professor of Neurology, Yale School of Medicine, for his assistance.
- Dr. Pierre N. Tariot and Dr. George T. Grossberg, authors: Memantine treatment in patients with moderate to severe Alzheimer disease already receiving donepezil: a randomized controlled trial. *JAMA*. 2004;291:317–324.

- Dr. Lawrence J. Hirsch, Chief of Division of Epilepsy and EEG, Yale School of Medicine, reviewer: A comparison of four treatments for generalized convulsive status epilepticus. *N Engl J Med.* 1998;339:792–798.
- Dr. Anthony G. Marson, first author: (1) The SANAD study of effectiveness of carbamazepine, gabapentin, lamotrigine, oxcarbazepine, or topiramate for treatment of partial epilepsy: an unblinded randomised controlled trial. *Lancet.* 2007;369:1000–1015; (2) The SANAD study of effectiveness of valproate, lamotrigine, or topiramate for generalised and unclassifiable epilepsy: an unblinded randomised controlled trial. Lancet. 2007;369:1016–1026.
- Dr. Michel D. Ferrari, corresponding author: Treatment of migraine attacks with sumatriptan. The subcutaneous sumatriptan international study group. *N Engl J Med.* 1991;325:316–321.
- Dr. Frank M. Sullivan, first author: Early treatment with prednisolone or acyclovir in Bell's palsy. *N Engl J Med.* 2007;357:1598–1607.
- Dr. Serena Spudich, Chief of Division of Neurological Infections and Global Neurology, Yale School of Medicine, reviewer:. Dexamethasone in adults with bacterial meningitis. *N Engl J Med.* 2002;347:1549–1556.
- Dr. Karl Kieburtz, co-author: Levodopa and the progression of Parkinson's disease. *N Engl J Med.* 2004;351:2498-2508.
- Dr. Günther Deuschl, first author: A randomized trial of deep-brain stimulation for Parkinson's disease. *N Engl J Med.* 2006;355:896–908.
- Dr. David Barnes, first author of: Barnes D, Hughes RA, Morris RW, Wade-Jones O, Brown P, Britton T, Francis DA, Perkin GD, Rudge P, Swash M, Katifi H, Farmer S, Frankel J. Randomised trial of oral and intravenous methylprednisolone in acute relapses of multiple sclerosis. *Lancet.* 1997;349:902-906.
- Dr. Roy W. Beck, co-author: Intramuscular interferon beta-1a therapy initiated during a first demyelinating event in multiple sclerosis. *N Engl J Med.* 2000;343:898–904. Also, first-author: A randomized, controlled trial of corticosteroids in the treatment of acute optic neuritis. *N Engl J Med.* 1992;326:581–588.
- Dr. Giancarlo Comi, first author: Effect of glatiramer acetate on conversion to clinically definite multiple sclerosis in patients with clinically isolated syndrome: a randomised, double-blind, placebo-controlled trial. *Lancet.* 2009;374:1503–1511. We also appreciate Dr. Natalia Ashtamker and Teva Pharmaceutical Industries Ltd. for their assistance.
- Dr. Alfred W. Sandrock, senior author: Natalizumab plus interferon beta-1a for relapsing multiple sclerosis. *N Engl J Med.* 2006;354:911–923.

- Dr. Jeffrey A. Cohen, first author: Oral fingolimod or intramuscular interferon for relapsing multiple sclerosis. *N Engl J Med.* 2010;362:402–415.
- Dr. Ralf Gold, first author: Placebo-controlled phase 3 study of oral BG-12 for relapsing multiple sclerosis. *N Engl J Med.* 2012;367:1098–1107.
- Dr. Robert J. Fox, first author: Placebo-controlled phase 3 study of oral BG-12 or glatiramer in multiple sclerosis. *N Engl J Med.* 2012;367:1087–1097
- Dr. Michael Holzer, co-author and guarantor: Mild therapeutic hypothermia to improve the neurologic outcome after cardiac arrest. *N Engl J Med.* 2002;346:549–556.
- Dr. Stephen A. Bernard, first author: Treatment of comatose survivors of out-of-hospital cardiac arrest with induced hypothermia. *N Engl J Med.* 2002;346:557–563.
- Dr. D. James Cooper and Dr. Jeffrey V. Rosenfeld, co-authors: Decompressive craniectomy in diffuse traumatic brain injury. *N Engl J Med.* 2011;364:1493–1502.
- Dr. George S. Allen, first author: Cerebral arterial spasm—a controlled trial of nimodipine in patients with subarachnoid hemorrhage. *N Engl J Med.* 1983;308:619–624.
- Dr. Richard A.C. Hughes and Dr. David R. Cornblath, writing committee members for: Randomised trial of plasma exchange, intravenous immunoglobulin, and combined treatments in Guillain-Barré syndrome. Plasma exchange/Sandoglobulin Guillain-Barré Syndrome Trial Group. *Lancet.* 1997;349:225–230.
- Dr. Vera Bril, senior author: Comparison of IVIg and PLEX in patients with myasthenia gravis. *Neurology.* 2011;76:2017–2023.
- Dr. Vincent Meininger, senior author: Bensimon G, Lacomblez L, Meininger V. A controlled trial of riluzole in amyotrophic lateral sclerosis. *N Engl J Med.* 1994;330:585–591.
- Dr. Joachim M. Baehring, Clinical Program Leader, Brain Tumor Program, Smilow Cancer Hospital, New Haven, CT, reviewer: (1) Radiotherapy plus concomitant and adjuvant temozolomide for glioblastoma. *N Engl J Med.* 2005;352:987–996. (2) MGMT gene silencing and benefit from temozolomide in glioblastoma. *N Engl J Med.* 2005;352:997–1003.
- Dr. Elias M. Michaelides, Assistant Professor of Surgery (Otolaryngology), and Dr. Dhasakumar S. Navaratnam, Associate Professor of Neurology and Neurobiology, Yale School of Medicine, reviewers: The canalith repositioning procedure: for treatment of benign paroxysmal positional vertigo. *Otolaryngo Head Neck Surg.* 1992;107:399–404. We also appreciate Cathryn Epley, President

of Vesticon (Portland, OR), for her assistance. We thank Michael T. Loscalzo for contributing the illustration accompanying the summary of this article.

- Dr. Sanjeev V. Kothare, Director of Pediatric Sleep Program, New York University Medical Center, reviewer: Randomized, double-blind, placebo-controlled crossover trial of modafinil in the treatment of excessive daytime sleepiness in narcolepsy. *Neurology.* 1997;49:444–451
- Dr. Claudia Trenkwalder, first author: Efficacy of rotigotine for treatment of moderate-to-severe restless legs syndrome: A randomised, double-blind, placebo-controlled trial. *Lancet Neurol.* 2008;7:595–604. We also appreciate Dr. Brian B. Koo, Director of the Sleep Medicine Program at the Connecticut Veterans Affairs Healthcare System, for his assistance.
- Dr. Wilco C. Peul, first author: Surgery versus prolonged conservative treatment for sciatica. *N Engl J Med.* 2007;356:2245–2256.
- Dr. James N. Weinstein, first author: Surgical versus nonsurgical treatment for lumbar degenerative spondylolisthesis. *N Engl J Med.* 2007;356:2257–2270
- Dr. Mark N. Hadley, Professor of Neurosurgery, The University of Alabama at Birmingham School of Medicine, reviewer: A randomized, controlled trial of methylprednisolone or naloxone in the treatment of acute spinal-cord injury. Results of the Second National Acute Spinal Cord Injury Study. *N Engl J Med.* 1990;322:1405–1411.
- Dr. John R. Marler, corresponding author: Tissue plasminogen activator for acute ischemic stroke. The National Institute of Neurological Disorders and Stroke rt-PA Stroke Study Group. *N Engl J Med.* 1995;333:1581–1587.
- Dr. Werner Hacke, first author: Thrombolysis with alteplase 3 to 4.5 hours after acute ischemic stroke. *N Engl J Med.* 2008;359:1317–1329.
- Dr. Anthony Furlan, first author: Intra-arterial prourokinase for acute ischemic stroke. The PROACT II study: A randomized controlled trial. Prolyse in Acute Cerebral Thromboembolism. *JAMA.* 1999;282:2003–2011.
- Dr. Joseph P. Broderick, first author: Endovascular therapy after intravenous t-PA versus t-PA alone for stroke. *N Engl J Med.* 2013;368:893–903.
- Dr. Chelsea S. Kidwell and Dr. Reza Jahan, co-authors: A trial of imaging selection and endovascular treatment for ischemic stroke. *N Engl J Med.* 2013;368:914–923.

- Dr. Seemant Chaturvedi, Professor of Neurology, University of Miami Miller School of Medicine, reviewer: (1) Beneficial effect of carotid endarterectomy in symptomatic patients with high-grade carotid stenosis. North American Symptomatic Carotid Endarterectomy Trial Collaborators. *N Engl J Med*. 1991;325:445–453. (2) Benefit of carotid endarterectomy in patients with symptomatic moderate or severe stenosis. North American Symptomatic Carotid Endarterectomy Trial Collaborators. *N Engl J Med*. 1998;339:1415–1425.
- Dr. Harold P. Adams, publications committee member for: Endarterectomy for asymptomatic carotid artery stenosis. Executive Committee for the Asymptomatic Carotid Atherosclerosis Study. *JAMA*. 1995;273:1421–1428.
- Dr. Zheng-Ming Chen, corresponding author of: CAST: Randomised placebo-controlled trial of early aspirin use in 20,000 patients with acute ischaemic stroke. CAST (Chinese Acute Stroke Trial) Collaborative Group. *Lancet*. 1997;349:1641–1649.
- Dr. Peter A. G. Sandercock, corresponding author of: The International Stroke Trial (IST): A randomised trial of aspirin, subcutaneous heparin, both, or neither among 19,435 patients with acute ischaemic stroke. International Stroke Trial Collaborative Group. *Lancet*. 1997;349:1569–1581.
- Professor Dr. Hans C. Diener, first author of: European Stroke Prevention Study. 2. Dipyridamole and acetylsalicylic acid in the secondary prevention of stroke. *J Neurol Sci*. 1996;143:1–13.
- Dr. K. Michael Welch, President and CEO of Rosalind Franklin University of Medicine and Science, North Chicago, IL, co-author: High-dose atorvastatin after stroke or transient ischemic attack. *N Engl J Med*. 2006;355:549–559.

CONTRIBUTORS

Hardik P. Amin, MD
Assistant Professor of Neurology
Yale School of Medicine
New Haven, Connecticut

Allison Arch, MD
Resident, Yale Neurology
Yale School of Medicine
New Haven, Connecticut

Mary A. Bailey, MD
Assistant Professor of Neurology
Yale School of Medicine
New Haven, Connecticut

Benjamin N. Blond, MD
Resident, Yale Neurology
Yale School of Medicine
New Haven, Connecticut

Daniel C. Brooks, MD
Resident, Yale Neurology
Yale School of Medicine
New Haven, Connecticut

Sarah E. Buckingham, MD
Resident, Yale Neurology
Yale School of Medicine
New Haven, Connecticut

Amy Chan, MD
Resident, Yale Neurology
Yale School of Medicine
New Haven, Connecticut

Robert J. Claycomb, MD, PhD
Resident, Yale Neurology
Yale School of Medicine
New Haven, Connecticut

Pue Farooque, DO
Assistant Professor of Neurology
Yale School of Medicine
New Haven, Connecticut

Shivani Ghoshal, MD
Resident, Yale Neurology
Yale School of Medicine
New Haven, Connecticut

Ryan A. Grant, MD, MS
Assistant Professor of Medicine
Frank Netter School of Medicine
Quinnipiac University
Resident, Yale Neurosurgery
Yale School of Medicine
New Haven, Connecticut

Abeer J. Hani, MD
Fellow, Clinical Neurophysiology
Duke University Medical Center
Durham, North Carolina

Matthew D. Kalp, MD
Fellow, Vascular Neurology
Duke University Medical Center
Durham, North Carolina

Luis Kolb, MD
Resident, Yale Neurosurgery
Yale School of Medicine
New Haven, Connecticut

Mark Landreneau, MD
Resident, Yale Neurology
Yale School of Medicine
New Haven, Connecticut

Joshua Lovinger, MD, MA
Fellow, Vascular Neurology
New York University School of Medicine
New York, New York

Brian Mac Grory, MB, BCh, BAO
Resident, Yale Neurology
Yale School of Medicine
New Haven, Connecticut

Sarah A. Mulukutla, MD, MPH
Resident, Yale Neurology
Yale School of Medicine
New Haven, Connecticut

Sacit Bulent Omay, MD
Resident, Yale Neurosurgery
Yale School of Medicine
New Haven, Connecticut

Ashish L. Ranpura, MD, PhD
Resident, Yale Neurology
New Haven, Connecticut

Kimberly R. Robeson, MD
Assistant Professor of Neurology
Yale School of Medicine
New Haven, Connecticut

Irene Hwa Yang, MD
Resident, Yale Neurology
New Haven, Connecticut

Teddy S. Youn, MD
Fellow, Division of Neurocritical Care and Emergency Neurology
Yale School of Medicine
New Haven, Connecticut

SECTION I

Behavioral Neurology

1

Cholinesterase Inhibitors for Alzheimer's Disease

ASHISH L. RANPURA

> These data indicate that donepezil is a well-tolerated drug that improves cognition and global function in patients with mild to moderate [Alzheimer's disease].
> —Rogers et al.[1]

Research Question: Does donepezil, an acetylcholinesterase (AChE) inhibitor with relatively high CNS specificity, improve cognitive and global functional outcomes in patients with Alzheimer's disease (AD)?[1]

Funding: Eisai Co., Ltd.

Year Study Began: 1993

Year Study Published: 1998

Study Location: 20 sites in the United States.

Who Was Studied: Men and women of any race aged ≥50 years and diagnosed with probable AD by NINCDS–ADRDA criteria, as well as patients diagnosed by DSM-III-R criteria (categories 290.00 or 290.10), with no clinical or laboratory evidence of a cause for their dementia other than AD.

The NINCDS–ADRDA (National Institute of Neurological and Communicative Disorders and Stroke–Alzheimer's Disease and Related Disorders Association) criteria for the diagnosis of probable AD are dementia established by examination and objective testing, with deficits in two or more cognitive areas, progressive worsening of memory and other cognitive functions, no disturbance of consciousness, and onset between the ages of 40 and 90.

The DSM-III-R (*Diagnostic and Statistical Manual of Mental Disorders*, 3rd ed. revised) criteria for dementia are (A) impairment in short- and long-term memory; (B) impairment in abstract thinking or judgement, or impairment of higher cortical functions or personality changes; and (C) evidence that the cognitive disturbance resulting from criteria (A) and (B) significantly interferes with work, usual social activities, or relationship with others. Symptoms do not occur exclusively during the course of delirium (D) and there is either (E1) evidence of a specific organic factor judged to be etiologically related to the disturbance, or (E2) in the absence of such evidence, an etiological factor can be presumed if the disturbance cannot be accounted for by any nonorganic mental disorder.

Who Was Excluded: Patients with insulin-dependent diabetes or other endocrine disorders; asthma or obstructive pulmonary disease; or clinically significant uncontrolled gastrointestinal, hepatic, or cardiovascular diseases. Patients were also excluded if they were known to be hypersensitive to AChE inhibitors, or if they had been taking tacrine or other investigational drugs for dementia within 1 month of the baseline assessment.

How Many Patients: 473

Study Overview: See Figure 1.1 for a summary of the trial's design.

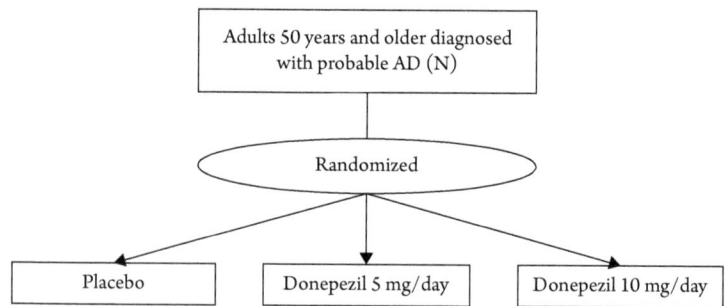

Figure 1.1 Summary of Rogers et al. Design.

Study Intervention: This was a randomized, double-blind, placebo-controlled trial, ending with a single-blind placebo washout. Patients received their treatment as a single dose, once each evening. There were 3 groups: placebo, lower dosage donepezil (5 mg/day), and maximum dosage donepazil (10 mg/day). For the maximum dosage group, a blinded forced-titration scheme was used in which the subjects received 5 mg/day for the first week, and then 10 mg/day thereafter.

Follow-Up: Measures of clinical outcomes were taken at baseline, and again at 6, 12, 18, and 24 weeks. A final measurement was taken after a 6-week posttherapeutic placebo washout. Patients completing the 24-week double-blind phase were eligible for continued treatment with donepezil in a subsequent open-label study.

Endpoints: Primary outcomes: change in the cognitive portion of the Alzheimer's Disease Assessment Scale (ADAS-Cog), and a Clinician's Interview-Based Impression of Change Plus Caregiver Input (CIBIC-Plus) at study endpoint. ADAS-Cog[2] scores range from 0–70, with higher scores (≥ 18) indicating impaired performance. Differences on the scale of at least 4 points are considered clinically meaningful, although the test may be biased to predict clinical decline more readily than improvement.[3] The CIBIC-Plus[4] is a global measure of detectable change in cognition, function, and behavior requiring separate interviews with patients and caregivers. It is scored as a 7-point categorical rating, with each item scored from 1 ("markedly improved"), to 4 ("no change"), and up to 7 ("markedly worse"). Total score range is therefore 7–49, with higher scores indicating clinical deterioration. Secondary outcomes: Changes in scores for the Mini-Mental State Examination (MMSE), a patient-rated quality of life measure (QoL), and the Clinical Dementia Rating scale Sum of Boxes (CDR-SB).

RESULTS

- CDR scores were used to characterize the patients during screening; 74%–76% of patients had a score of 1 (mild dementia), and 25% had a score of 2 (moderate dementia). The baseline degree of impairment was not statistically different between the treatment and placebo arms.
- The mean ADAS-Cog score for the placebo group improved after 6 weeks, then steadily worsened.

- There was a statistically significant improvement in ADAS-Cog scores in the treatment arm versus placebo (see Table 1.1). There was dose-dependency in the treatment effect of donepezil.
- Similarly, CIBIC-Plus ratings showed more therapeutic success in the treatment arm compared to the placebo arm (see Table 1.1).
- There were dose-dependent improvements in MMSE scores, and dose-independent stabilization of CDR-SB scores (for MMSE scores, the drug–placebo difference was 1.21 and 1.36 at 5 mg/day and 10 mg/day, respectively; for CDR-SB scores, the drug–placebo difference was 0.59 and 0.60 at 5 mg/day and 10 mg/day, respectively; all P values < 0.001). Patient-rated QoL measures did not significantly differ between groups.
- After the 6-week washout period, scores in the treatment arms could no longer be statistically differentiated from scores in the placebo arm, suggesting that the benefits conferred by donepezil relied on its continued administration. There was no clinical rebound or delayed exacerbation of symptoms in the treatment arm after withdrawal of the medication.
- High-dose donepezil was associated with more frequent transient adverse effects, including fatigue, diarrhea, nausea, vomiting, and muscle cramps, consistent with the drug's cholinergic activity.

Table 1.1. SUMMARY OF THE TRIAL'S KEY FINDINGS

	Placebo	Donepezil 5 mg/day	Donepezil 10 mg/day
Mean ADAS-Cog change	1.82 ± 0.49	−0.67 ± 0.51	−1.06 ± 0.51
% of patients with progression of symptoms (ADAS-Cog change ≥ 0)	42.3	20.3	18.9
Mean CIBIC-Plus	4.51 ± 0.08	4.15 ± 0.09	4.07 ± 0.07
% of patients with clinical improvement (CIBIC-Plus ≤ 3)	11	26	25
Drug–placebo difference for ADAS-Cog		−2.49 ($P < 0.0001$)	−2.88 ($P < 0.0001$)
Drug–placebo difference for CIBIC-Plus		0.36 ($P = 0.0047$)	0.44 ($P < 0.0001$)

Criticisms and Limitations: The study population of "young old" patients suffering from dementia without any medical comorbidities may not have adequately represented real-world AD patients. In practice, the benefits of donepezil must be weighed against its cholinergic side effects and its interactions with other medications. Additionally, the mean changes in ADAS-Cog scores were in the range of 1–2 points, far less than the 4-point threshold usually held to represent clinically meaningful effects. Mean CIBIC-Plus scores improved, but still hovered around 4, which may not represent a significant clinical change over the duration of the study. It is also generally felt that MMSE scores that differ by <3 points are functionally equivalent. Furthermore, it is not clear that cognitive change as measured by ADAS-Cog and the MMSE is predictive of disability, the need for institutionalization, or overall morbidity. Finally, patients did not have clinical follow-up after the completion of the 30-week observation period. Given the progressive nature of AD, it is unclear whether the effects of donepezil therapy are durable.

Other Relevant Studies and Information:

- A 1-year trial conducted in Norway showed similar and durable effects during continued administration.[5] More data are needed to determine the appropriate duration of donepezil therapy.
- Newer AChE inhibitors such as rivastigmine and galantamine have shown similar efficacy to donepezil, with only minor variations in their side effect profiles.[6]
- The cost-effectiveness of long-term donepezil treatment has been questioned.[7]
- Current guidelines for the use of donepezil in the mild to moderate stages of Alzheimer's disease recommend a starting dose of 5 mg nightly for 1 month, increasing to 10 mg nightly thereafter as tolerated.

Summary and Implications: This randomized clinical trial demonstrated that 5 and 10 mg daily donepezil effectively slowed the cognitive decline associated with AD for up to 6 months in a dose-dependent fashion; however, the absolute benefits were modest. The long-term utility of donepezil for treatment of AD remains in question, as the medication does not alter the ultimate course of the disease.

CLINICAL CASE: CHOLINESTERASE INHIBITORS IN ALZHEIMER'S DISEASE

Case History:
A 69-year-old right-handed gentleman visits your clinic with his wife, complaining of increasing difficulty concentrating in the last few months. His wife tells you that the patient retired from his job as a real estate manager a few years earlier than he would have liked because he was having trouble making financial decisions and had started to forget important information about his clients. She feels that her husband's early retirement has left him depressed; he has become more socially withdrawn and has given up his weekly game of golf. During your examination, you notice that whenever he is questioned directly, the patient turns to his wife for help in answering. He achieves a score of 18/30 on a bedside MMSE, with errors scored in orientation, concentration, recall, language, and figure drawing. The neurological exam is otherwise unremarkable.

MRI of the brain shows mild diffuse cortical volume loss, with a few punctuate T2-weighted hyperintensities in the periventricular white matter bilaterally. Glucose, vitamin B_{12}, TSH, electrolytes, and LFTs are all within normal limits. RPR and HIV testing is negative. In the absence of other explanations, you feel that AD is the best diagnosis. How would you proceed with treatment?

Suggested Answer:
Having ruled out reversible causes of dementia, the diagnosis of AD is reasonable in these circumstances. Depression is often a significant comorbidity, and should be evaluated and treated independently. Among cholinesterase inhibitors, donepezil, rivastigmine, and galantamine are similar in efficacy and side effect profiles, but donepezil is generally the most cost effective.

It is important to warn patients about cholinergic side effects including nausea, GI upset, diarrhea, and fatigue. These side effects are the most common cause of noncompliance and treatment failure. Donepezil can be started at 5 mg PO daily for 4–6 weeks, with an increase to 10 mg PO daily if tolerated.

The goal of treatment is to slow or delay clinical deterioration, and expectations should be set carefully; treatment will not return the patient to their premorbid functional capacity. Caregivers will need education and support. Nonpharmacological interventions such as exercise and increased socialization play a critical role in retaining functional capacity.

References

1. Rogers SL, Farlow MR, Doody RS. A 24-week, double-blind, placebo-controlled trial of donepezil in patients with Alzheimer's disease. *Neurology*. 1998;50(1):136–145.
2. Rosen WG, Mohs RC, Davis KL. A new rating scale for Alzheimer's disease. *Am J Psychiatry*. 1984;141(11):1356–1364.
3. Rockwood K, Fay S, Gorman M, Carver D, Grahame JE. The clinical meaningfulness of ADAS-Cog changes in Alzheimer's disease patients treated with donepezil in an open-label trial. *BMC Neurol*. 2007;7:26.
4. Schneider LS, Olin JT, Doody RS, et al. Validity and reliability of the Alzheimer's Disease Cooperative Study-Clinical Global Impression of Change. The Alzheimer's Disease Cooperative Study. *Alzheimer Dis Assoc Disord*. 1997;11(suppl 2):S22–S32.
5. Winblad B, Engedal K, Soininen H, et al. (Donepezil Nordic Study Group). A 1-year, randomized, placebo-controlled study of donepezil in patients with mild to moderate AD. *Neurol*. 2001;57(3):489–495.
6. Bikrs, J. Cholinesterase inhibitors for Alzheimer's disease. *Cochrane Database Syst Rev*. 2006;1:CD005593.
7. Courtney C, Farrell D, Gray R, et al. (AD2000 Collaborative Group). Long-term donepezil treatment in 565 patients with Alzheimer's disease (AD2000): randomised double-blind trial. *Lancet*. 2004;363(9427):2105–2115.

2

Memantine for Alzheimer's Disease

JOSHUA LOVINGER

> In patients with moderate to severe AD receiving stable doses of donepezil, memantine resulted in significantly better outcomes than placebo on measures of cognition, activities of daily living, global outcome, and behavior and was well-tolerated.[1]
>
> —Tariot et al.

Research Question: Memantine, an NMDA-receptor antagonist, has shown efficacy in patients with moderate to severe Alzheimer's disease (AD) as a monotherapy. Is there clinical benefit to initiation of memantine in patients with moderate to severe AD already on the cholinesterase inhibitor donepezil?[1]

Funding: Forest Laboratories.

Year Study Began: 2001

Year Study Published: 2004

Study Location: 37 US sites.

Who Was Studied: Patients who had a diagnosis of probable AD, according to the National Institute of Neurological and Communicative Disorders and Stroke–Alzheimer's Disease and Related Disorders Association (NINCDS-ADRDA) criteria (Box 2.1)[2]:

Box 2.1 NINCDS-ADRDA CRITERIA FOR DIAGNOSIS OF PROBABLE ALZHEIMER'S DISEASE

1. Dementia is established by clinical examination and neuropsychological tests
2. Deficits in two or more areas of cognition
3. Progressive worsening of memory and other cognitive functions
4. No disturbance of consciousness
5. Onset between ages 40 and 90, most often after age 65
6. Absence of systemic disorders or other brain diseases that in and of themselves could account for the progressive deficits in memory and cognition

---

Inclusion criteria were as follows: Mini-Mental State Examination (MMSE)[3] score of 5 to 14 at both screening and baseline; minimum age of 50 years; a recent MRI or CT scan (within 12 months) consistent with a diagnosis of probable AD; ongoing cholinesterase inhibitor therapy with donepezil for more than 6 months before entrance into the trial and at a stable dose (5-10 mg/d) for at least 3 months; a knowledgeable and reliable caregiver to accompany the patient to research visits and oversee the administration of the investigational agent during the trial; residence in the community; ambulatory or ambulatory-aided (ie, walker or cane) ability; and stable medical condition. Patients were permitted to continue receiving stable doses of concomitant medications, including antidepressants, antihypertensives, anti-inflammatory drugs, atypical antipsychotics, antiparkinsonian drugs, anticoagulants, laxatives, diuretics, and sedatives/hypnotics.[4]

Who Was Excluded: "Patients were excluded for clinically significant [vitamin] B_{12} or folate deficiency; active pulmonary, gastrointestinal, renal, hepatic, endocrine, or cardiovascular disease; other psychiatric or central nervous system disorders; computed tomographic or magnetic resonance imaging evidence of clinically significant central nervous system disorders other than probable

AD; dementia complicated by other organic disease; or a modified Hachinski Ischemia Score [Table 2.1] of more than 4 at screening"[5] (to exclude patients with presumed vascular dementia).

Table 2.1. CLINICAL FEATURES OF THE MODIFIED HACHINSKI ISCHEMIC SCORE[a]

Feature	Point value
Abrupt onset	2
Stepwise deterioration	1
Somatic complaints	1
Emotional incontinence	1
History or presence of hypertension	1
History of strokes	2
Focal neurologic symptoms	2
Focal neurologic signs	2

[a] Scores of 0–2 are more consistent with primary neurodegenerative disease (e.g., AD). Scores ≥4 are more consistent with multi-infarct (vascular) dementia. The Ischemic Score does *not* differentiate between patients with multi-infarct dementia alone and patients with both disorders (multi-infarct dementia *and* a primary neurodegenerative disease).

Rosen WG, Terry RD, Fuld PA, Katzman R, Peck A. Pathological verification of Ischemic Score in differentiation of dementias. *Ann Neurol*. 1980;7(5):486–488. For the original Ischemic Score, with 13 rather than 8 items: Hachinski VC, Illff LD, Zilhka E, et al. Cerebral blood flow in dementia. *Arch Neurol*. 1975;32(9):632–637. Both studies suffer from small sample numbers (Hachinski et al., N = 24; Rosen et al., N = 14). Hachinski et al.'s study included relatively young patients (some were in their 40s and 50s; the eldest was 73); in Rosen et al.'s study, the youngest patient was 74. The latter was a retrospective study and the Ischemic Score was calculated from review of patient records. There are more recent diagnostic criteria for vascular dementia (some utilizing imaging); e.g., Román GC, Tatemichi TK, Erkinjuntti T, et al. Vascular dementia: diagnostic criteria for research studies. Report of the NINDS-AIREN International Workshop. *Neurol*. 1993;43(2):250–260. See Pohjasvaara T, Mäntylä R, Ylikoski R, Kaste M, Erkinjuntti T. Comparison of different clinical criteria (DSM-III, ADDTC, ICD-10, NINDS-AIREN, DSM-IV) for the diagnosis of vascular dementia. National Institute of Neurological Disorders and Stroke-Association Internationale pour la Recherche et l'Enseignement en Neurosciences. *Stroke*. 2000;31(12):2952–2957.

How Many Patients: 404

Study Overview: See Figure 2.1 for a summary of the trial's design.

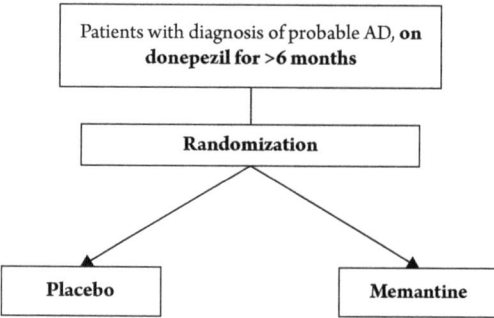

Figure 2.1 Summary of the Study's Design.

Study Intervention: Patients in the memantine group received memantine, "titrated in 5 mg weekly increments from a starting dose of 5 mg/d to 20 mg/d" (administered as 10 mg twice daily) by the beginning of week 4. From weeks 3–8, "transient dose adjustments of memantine treatment were permitted for patients experiencing dose-limiting adverse events. All patients receiving memantine were required to receive the target dose of 20 mg/d by the end of week 8."[5] Patients in the placebo group received placebo tablets that were visually identical to memantine. All patients were to maintain stable donepezil therapy at entry dose as prescribed by the patient's physician for the duration of the study.

Follow-Up: 24 weeks.

Endpoints: Primary endpoints included both cognitive and functional assessments: (1) Change from baseline on the Severe Impairment Battery (SIB) and (2) change from baseline on the modified 19-item AD Cooperative Study–Activities of Daily Living Inventory (ADCS-ADL$_{19}$), both at week 24. Secondary endpoints: (1) Clinician's Interview-Based Impression of Change Plus Caregiver Input (CIBIC-Plus), (2) Neuropsychiatric Inventory (NPI), (3) Behavioral Rating Scale for Geriatric Patients (BGP).

RESULTS

- Both cognitive and functional outcomes were better in the memantine versus placebo group (see Table 2.2).
- Memantine and placebo groups did not differ substantially in adverse effects; in fact, there was more treatment discontinuation due to adverse events in the placebo group. However, there was an increased incidence in confusion and headache in the memantine group (both occurring at more than twice the rate of the placebo group).[6]

Table 2.2. SUMMARY OF KEY FINDINGS FOR PRIMARY ENDPOINTS

Outcome Measure	Change from Baseline[a]					
	Endpoint (LOCF)[b]			Among Patients Who Made Week 24 Visit		
	Placebo	Memantine	P value	Placebo	Memantine	P value
SIB[c]	−2.5	0.9	<0.001	−2.4	1.0	<0.001
ADCS-ADL$_{19}$[d]	−3.4	−2.0	0.03	−3.3	−1.7	0.02

[a] Values are least squares mean scores.
[b] LOCF = last observation carried forward.
[c] SIB range of possible scores: 0–100. Higher score indicates better function.
[d] ADCS-ADL$_{19}$ range of possible scores: 0–54. Higher score indicates better function.

Criticisms and Limitations: The results of the trial are restricted to patients with MMSE scores of 5–14. Use of memantine alone or in combination with cholinesterase inhibitors in milder degrees of AD was not addressed in this study.[7]

The trial may have included a population with heterogeneous pathology.[8] While using the Ischemic Score to exclude patients with vascular dementia, it may have included patients with non-AD dementias. For example, the trial did not exclude patients on medications for parkinsonism.[9] The response of patients with severe dementia to memantine may differ between underlying etiologies of dementia.[10]

A high[11] percentage of patients discontinued study participation (fully a fourth of the placebo group, 51/201; and 30/203 assigned to receive memantine), which may have introduced inaccuracies in findings. However, in an older population with advanced dementia, this level of study dropouts is not unexpected.[12]

Though more patents in the placebo arm discontinued participation in the study prematurely because of adverse effects,[13] in the treatment arm the rate of confusion was almost quadruple that of the placebo arm (7.9% vs 2.0%).[14]

Other Relevant Studies and Information:

- A number of trials have since examined the role of memantine in more specific subgroups with dementia. Memantine did not show benefit for patients with Parkinson's disease dementia, adults with Down syndrome, or in frontotemporal lobar degeneration (FTLD). In one study, patients with dementia with Lewy bodies on memantine showed improved NPI scores compared to those receiving placebo.[15]
- This study complements the earlier one of Reisberg et al. that demonstrated the benefit of memantine monotherapy in patients with moderate to severe AD.[16] The results of this study are limited to patients

with moderate to severe AD; memantine has not shown benefit for mild AD.[7]
- Some subsequent studies have questioned the benefit of combination therapy over monotherapy.[17] One later study that did not show benefit to the combination of cholinesterase inhibitors and memantine included patients with MMSE scores between 10–22, which, while overlapping the population in Tariot et al. (MMSE = 5–14), included patients with *mild* AD as well.[18] A more recent trial adding extended-release memantine[19] in patients with moderate to severe AD already on donepezil replicated the positive findings regarding combination therapy of Tariot et al.[20]

Summary and Implications: In patients with severe AD on a stable dose of donepezil, the addition of memantine was better than placebo in improving cognitive outcomes and decreasing rate of functional decline.

CLINICAL CASE: MEMANTINE FOR ALZHEIMER'S DISEASE PATIENTS ALREADY ON DONEPEZIL

Case History:
A 75-year-old woman has been noted by her family to have a slowly progressive cognitive decline, which began with short-term memory loss. She now has marked limitation in her ability to perform activities of daily living and can no longer live alone. She does not have a history of stroke or focal neurologic symptoms. A workup did not reveal systemic or brain diseases to account for her memory loss. Her primary physician starts her on donepezil for presumed AD.

She is referred to you for evaluation. No history of psychosis is reported by her caregivers. She scores 0/3 on recall testing at 5 minutes. She has no tremor, rigidity, bradykinesia, or retropulsion on examination. She scores a 10 on the MMSE. Based upon the results of Tariot et al., how should this patient be treated?

Suggested Answer:
Tariot et al. showed that the addition of memantine, for a patient on a stable dose of donepezil, is well-tolerated. In patients with moderate to severe dementia, the addition of memantine to donepezil improved cognitive performance and slowed functional decline. It would be reasonable to proceed with a trial of combination therapy, adding memantine to her treatment regimen, while monitoring for clinical improvement or decreased rate of decline, as well as for potential side effects.[21]

References / Additional Footnotes

1. Tariot PN, Farlow MR, Grossberg GT et al. Memantine treatment in patients with moderate to severe Alzheimer disease already receiving donepezil: a randomized controlled trial. *JAMA.* 2004;291(3):317–324.
2. "A diagnosis of *definite* Alzheimer's disease requires histopathologic confirmation. A clinical diagnosis of *possible* Alzheimer's disease may be made in the presence of other significant diseases, particularly if, on clinical judgment, Alzheimer's disease is considered the more likely cause of the progressive dementia. The clinical diagnosis of *possible*, rather than *probable* Alzheimer's disease may be used if the presentation or the course is somewhat aberrant." McKhann G, Drachman D, Folstein M, et al. Clinical diagnosis of Alzheimer's Disease: report of the NINCDS-ADRDA Work Group under the auspices of Department of Health and Human Services Task Force on Alzheimer's Disease. *Neurology.* 1984;34(7):939–944. For revision of these criteria: McKhann GM, Knopman DS, Chertkow H, et al. The diagnosis of dementia due to Alzheimer's disease: recommendations from the National Institute on Aging-Alzheimer's Association workgroups on diagnostic guidelines for Alzheimer's disease. *Alzheimers Dement.* 2011;7(3):263–269. In 1998 NINCDS was renamed the National Institute of Neurological Disorders and Stroke (NINDS)—its current name.
3. Folstein MF, Folstein SE, McHugh PR. "Mini-mental state." A practical method for grading the cognitive state of patients for the clinician. *J Psychiatr Res.* 1975;12(3):189–198.
4. Tariot et al., p. 318. Contrast Reisberg B, Doody R, Stöffler A, et al. Memantine in moderate-to-severe Alzheimer's disease. *NEJM.* 2003;348(14):1333–1341. There, patients receiving antiparkinsonian agents, hypnotic or anxiolytic agents, and antipsychotic (neuroleptic) agents were excluded. Patients on antiparkinsonian agents would typically be excluded from more recent AD trials.
5. Tariot et al., p. 318.
6. Tariot et al., p. 320. A higher incidence of headache was also seen in a trial of extended-release memantine at a higher dose (28 mg daily), though not to the degree see in Tariot et al. See Grossberg GT, Manes F, Allegri RF, et al. The safety, tolerability, and efficacy of once-daily memantine (28 mg): a multinational, randomized, double-blind, placebo-controlled trial in patients with moderate-to-severe Alzheimer's disease taking cholinesterase inhibitors. *CNS Drugs.* 2013;27(6):469–478. The prevalence of headache was only 5.6% versus 5.1% toward the group receiving memantine. A significant increase in the rate of confusion was *not* seen in the group receiving memantine.
7. See, e.g., Schneider LS, Dagerman KS, Higgins JP, McShane R. Lack of evidence for the efficacy of memantine in mild Alzheimer disease. Arch Neurol. 2011;68(8):991–998.
8. Obtaining a "pure AD" population may not often be feasible as, even using strict clinical criteria for AD, a proportion of people meeting these may have no AD pathology at autopsy or mixed pathology. Many trials for dementia then end up including patients with heterogeneous pathology.
9. The trial of Reisberg et al. did exclude patients on medications for parkinsonism. Though in our trial the number of patients on these was <20%, this does not preclude a proportion of patients with dementia related to Parkinson disease or dementia with Lewy bodies.
10. Memantine has now been studied specifically in patients with dementia with Lewy bodies and Parkinson disease dementia: (1) Aarsland D, Ballard C, Walker Z,

et al. Memantine in patients with Parkinson's disease dementia or dementia with Lewy bodies: a double-blind, placebo-controlled, multicentre trial. *Lancet Neurol.* 2009;8(7):613–618; (2) Emre M, Tsolaki M, Bonuccelli U, et al. Memantine for patients with Parkinson's disease dementia or dementia with Lewy bodies: a randomised, double-blind, placebo-controlled trial. *Lancet Neurol.* 2010;9(10):969–977.

11. The AAN's evidence classification criteria include study completion rates; studies with completion rates below 80% are downgraded.
12. The prior trial of memantine monotherapy in patients with moderate-to-severe AD also had both a high exclusion rate and a high dropout rate. See Rikkert MG, Dekkers WJ, Scheltens P, Verhey F. Memantine in moderate-to-severe Alzheimer disease evidence and ethics based? *Alzheimer Dis Assoc Disord.* 2004;18(1):47–48. For a discussion of study dropout rates and introduction of error using LOCF, see Prakash A, Risser RC, Mallinckrodt CH. The impact of analytic method on interpretation of outcomes in longitudinal clinical trials. *Int J Clin Pract.* 2008;62(8):1147–1158. Using the LOCF method, the last score on SIB of the patient who dropped out of the trial would be carried forward and assumed to be the score for the final data point.
13. Which might be construed as arguing for a favorable drug effect.
14. Tariot et al., p. 320.
15. For studies on PDD and DLB, see note 9. Hanney M, Prasher V, Williams N, et al. Memantine for dementia in adults older than 40 years with Down's syndrome (MEADOWS): a randomised, double-blind, placebo-controlled trial. *Lancet.* 2012;379(9815):528–536. For FTLD (for this study, behavioral variant FTD or semantic dementia): Boxer AL, Knopman DS, Kaufer DI, et al. Memantine in patients with frontotemporal lobar degeneration: a multicentre, randomised, double-blind, placebo-controlled trial. *Lancet Neurol.* 2013;12(2):149–156.
16. See Reisberg et al. The most recent American Academy of Neurology guidelines for management of dementia predate the clinical introduction of memantine and donepezil. Doody RS, Stevens JC, Beck C, et al. Practice parameter: management of dementia (an evidence-based review). Report of the Quality Standards Subcommittee of the American Academy of Neurology. *Neurology.* 2001;56(9):1154–1166.
17. E.g., Howard R., McShane R, Lindesay J., et al. Donepezil and memantine for moderate-to-severe Alzheimer's disease. *N Engl J Med.* 2012;366(10):893–903. The MMSE scores for inclusion here were 5–13.
18. Multiple types of cholinesterase inhibitors were included (donepezil, rivastigmine, galantamine) and, as noted, the MMSE range included both moderate and *mild* AD (memantine has not shown benefit for the mild group in multiple studies). See Porsteinsson AP, Grossberg GT, Mintzer J, Olin JT; Memantine MEM-MD-12 Study Group. Memantine treatment in patients with mild to moderate Alzheimer's disease already receiving a cholinesterase inhibitor: a randomized, double-blind, placebo-controlled trial. *Curr Alzheimer Res.* 2008;5(1):83–89.
19. At a dose of 28 mg daily, rather than 10 mg twice daily used in the trial in Tariot et al.
20. In addition, no increase in confusion was seen in the memantine group; Grossberg et al. (MMSE scores: 3–14.)
21. Especially since the absolute benefit of the addition of memantine is small, the population with dementia is already at higher risk for delirium (and the study in Tariot et al. saw an increased incidence of confusion with memantine use—though this was not seen in Grossberg et al.), and, when possible, polypharmacy in the elderly should be avoided.

SECTION II

Epilepsy

3

Lorazepam for Generalized Status Epilepticus

PUE FAROOQUE

Although lorazepam was no more efficacious than phenobarbital or than diazepam and phenytoin, it is easier to use.
—Treiman et al.[1]

Research Question: What is the best initial drug treatment for generalized status epilepticus?[1]

Funding: Department of Veterans Affairs Medical Research Service Cooperative Studies Program (CSP 265).

Year Study Began: 1990

Year Study Published: 1998

Study Location: 16 Veterans Affairs medical centers and 6 affiliated university hospitals in the United States.

Who Was Studied: All patients who presented to the hospital with either overt or subtle generalized convulsive status epilepticus at the time of evaluation regardless of prior drug treatment from July 1990 to June 1995. "Overt generalized convulsive status epilepticus was defined as recurrent (two or more) convulsions without complete recovery between seizures or continuous convulsive activity for more than 10 minutes and subtle generalized convulsive status as the stage of generalized status epilepticus when the patient is in continuous coma with ictal discharges seen on electroencephalogram (EEG) with or without subtle motor convulsions such as rhythmic muscle twitches or tonic eye deviation."[1]

Who Was Excluded: Status epilepticus of a type other than generalized convulsive; age <18 years; pregnancy; neurologic emergency requiring immediate surgical intervention; and the presence of a specific contraindication to therapy with hydantoin, benzodiazepines, or barbiturates. Patients were only allowed to be enrolled once, and if they received treatment and the seizures stopped they were not eligible for the study.

How Many Patients: 570

Study Overview: See Figure 3.1 for a summary of the study design.

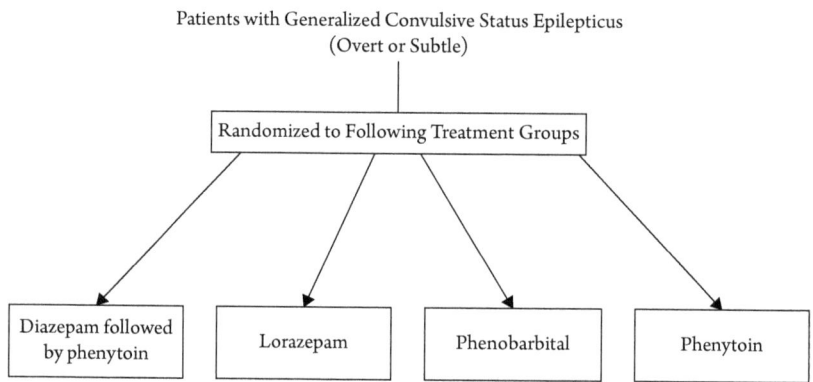

Figure 3.1 Summary of Study Design.

Study Intervention: Patients were classified as having either overt generalized status epilepticus or subtle status epilepticus and then were randomized to receive one of the following medications in a double-blind fashion: diazepam followed by phenytoin, lorazepam alone, phenobarbital alone, or phenytoin alone.

Follow-Up: Up to 30 days.

Endpoints: Primary outcome: Treatment was considered successful when all clinical and electrographic seizure activity ceased within 20 minutes after beginning the drug infusion and there was no return of seizure activity during the next 40 minutes.

Secondary outcome: Patients were monitored for 12 hours afterwards, both clinically and electrographically with EEG recording. Incidence of adverse reactions, hospitalization status, and mortality at 30 days were also obtained.

RESULTS

- Overall, the first treatment regime was successful in 55.5% of patients with overt status epilepticus and 14.9% of those with subtle status epilepticus. A low rate of efficacy was seen with the addition of the second medication regardless of which medication was used (Table 3.1).
- Lorazepam was effective significantly more often than phenytoin in patients with overt status epilepticus; however, no significant efficacy difference was seen between lorazepam and the other medications.
- Eleven percent of patients had recurrence of successfully treated status epilepticus within 12 hours; however, there were no significant differences in the rates of recurrence seen among the four treatment groups.
- Outcomes at 30 days were significantly worse for patients with subtle status epilepticus, with only 8.8% of the patients being discharged from the hospital in comparison to 50.1% of the overt status epilepticus patients. No significant differences in outcomes at 30 days were seen among the four treatment groups. Response to initial drug treatment was associated with better prognosis.
- Adverse effects were similar in all arms of the study.

Table 3.1. SUMMARY OF SUCCESSFUL TREATMENT IN EACH OF THE MEDICATION REGIMES

	Diazepam followed by Phenytoin	Lorazepam	Phenobarbital	Phenytoin
Overt Status Epilepticus	55.8% (95)	64.9% (97)	58.2% (91)	43.6% (101)
Subtle Status Epilepticus	8.3% (36)	17.9% (39)	24.2% (33)	7.7% (26)

Criticism and Limitations: There are limited controlled clinical trials for the treatment of status epilepticus, largely due to the difficulty of conducting such trials. Given the life-threatening nature of this emergent disorder, placebo-controlled trials are unethical. Thus those controlled trials that have been carried out have compared drugs already in use for the treatment of status epilepticus or have been given as prehospital treatment where this was not the standard of practice.[2] This study was the largest and a landmark comparative trial of antiseizure medications for the treatment of status epilepticus. However, this study only evaluated generalized status epilepticus; it did not include focal or refractory status epilepticus, and only had a limited number of patients with nonconvulsive status epilepticus.

Other Relevant Studies and Information:

- Lorazepam is the drug of choice for IV administration for treatment of convulsive status epilepticus.[3]
- No statistically significant difference between phenobarbital and a combination of diazepam and phenytoin was found in the treatment of status epilepticus.[4]
- In a prehospital treatment study, lorazepam was not significantly superior to diazepam; however, both medications were superior to placebo in controlling seizures and both decreased the chance of respiratory failure by 50% when compared to placebo.[2,5]
- In children, lorazepam has been found equally effective as diazepam followed by phenytoin.[6]
- A study evaluating prehospital treatment of status epilepticus by paramedics found intramuscular midazolam to be superior in controlling seizures versus intravenous lorazepam.[7]

Summary and Implications: Lorazepam has been shown as either equally or more efficacious in the treatment of status epilepticus versus other medications. Given its easier use, it is preferred as first-line treatment for status epilepticus.

CLINICAL CASE: INITIAL TREATMENT OF OVERT GENERALIZED STATUS EPILEPTICUS

Case History:
A 25-year-old right-handed male with known history of epilepsy presents to the emergency room with continuous generalized tonic-clonic seizures in the setting of having missed dosages of medication. His home medication is levetiracetam. Basic metabolic profile and CBC were unrevealing. Based on this study, what would be your first step?

Suggested Answer:
Based on this study the initial treatment should be lorazepam. Although there was no difference in benefit seen between lorazepam versus diazepam followed by phenytoin versus phenobarbital versus phenytoin alone, lorazepam would be recommended for its ease of use. This patient was typical of the patients enrolled in the trial. Of note, there have been no controlled trials with levetiracetam as the initial treatment in status epilepticus.

References

1. Treiman D et al. A comparison of four treatments for generalized convulsive status epilepticus. Veterans Affairs Status Epilepticus Cooperative Study Group. *N Engl J Med*. 1998;339(12):792–798.
2. Lockey A. Emergency department drug therapy for status epilepticus in adults. *Emerg Med J*. 2002;19:96–100.
3. Brophy G, Bell R, Claassen J, Alldredge B, et al. Guidelines for the evaluation and management of status epilepticus. *Neurocritcal Care*. 2012;17(1):3–23.
4. Shaner DM, McCurdy SA, Herring MO, Gabor AJ. Treatment of status epilepticus: a prospective comparison of diazepam and phenytoin versus phenobarbital and optional phenytoin. *Neurology*. 1988;38:202–207.
5. Alldredge BK, Gelb AM, Isaacs SM, et al. A comparison of lorazepam, diazepam, and placebo for the treatment of out-of-hospital status epilepticus. *N Engl J Med*. 2001;345(9):631–637.
6. Sreenath TG, Gupta P, Sharma KK, Krishnamurthy S. Lorazepam versus diazepam-phenytoin combination in the treatment of convulsive status epilepticus in children: a randomized controlled trial. *Eur J Paediatr Neurol*. 2010;14(2): 162–168.
7. Silbergleit R, Lowenstein D, Durkalski V, Conwit R; Neurological Emergency Treatment Trials (NETT) Investigators. RAMPART (Rapid Anticonvulsant Medication Prior to Arrival Trial): a double-blind randomized clinical trial of the efficacy of intramuscular midazolam versus intravenous lorazepam in the prehospital treatment of status epilepticus by paramedics. *Epilepsia*. 2011;52(suppl 8):45–47.

4

Lamotrigine for Partial Epilepsy

Arm A of the SANAD Trial

AMY CHAN

Lamotrigine is clinically better than carbamazepine, the standard drug treatment, for time to treatment failure outcomes *and is therefore a* cost-effective alternative *for patients diagnosed with partial onset seizures.* (emphasis added)

—MARSON ET AL.[1]

Research Question: What is the effectiveness of the newer anti-epileptic drugs against partial-onset seizures compared to carbamazepine, the widely accepted drug of first choice?[1]

Funding: The UK National Health Service Health Technology Assessment Programme, with an additional 20% of resources from companies with products assessed.

Year Study Began: 1999

Year Study Published: 2007

Study Location: Multiple hospital-based outpatient clinics in the United Kingdom

Who Was Studied: Patients aged >4 years with a history of 2 or more clinically definite unprovoked epileptic seizures in the previous year *and* for whom carbamazepine was deemed the better standard treatment option compared with valproate. These included patients who had

- newly diagnosed epilepsy,
- failed previous monotherapy treatment outside of randomization drugs, or
- had a period of remission but relapsed after withdrawal of treatment.

Who Was Excluded: Patients with acute symptomatic seizures only, were aged ≤4 years, or had a history of progressive neurological disease.

How Many Patients: 1,721

Study Overview: See Figure 4.1 for a summary of the trial's design.

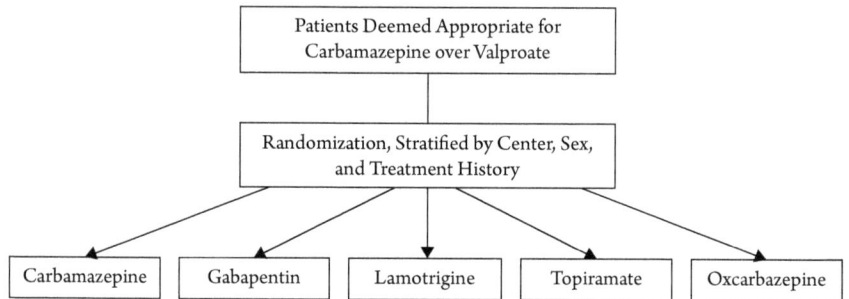

Figure 4.1 Summary of the Trial's Design.

Study Intervention: After a patient was randomized to one of the 5 study medications, the treating clinician, aided by guidelines, decided the rate of titration, initial maintenance dose, and any subsequent increments or decrements. The goal was to control seizures with a minimum effective dose of drug as assigned.

Follow-Up: 3 months, 6 months, 1 year, and at successive yearly intervals thereafter. Patients were followed up according to the principle of intention to treat.

Endpoints: Primary outcomes: (1) time from randomization to treatment failure, and (2) time from randomization to achievement of a 1-year remission. Secondary outcomes: (1) time from randomization to first seizure, (2) time to achieve a 2-year remission, (3) incidence of clinically important adverse events and side effects, and (4) quality of life outcomes and cost-effectiveness.

RESULTS

- Full dose range was explored for all treatment arms before accepting treatment failure.
- There was a statistically significant benefit, as measured by time to treatment failure, of lamotrigine (LTG) over carbamazepine (CBZ) (HR = 0.78; 95% CI 0.63–0.97), gabapentin (GBP) (HR 0.65; 95% CI 0.52–0.80), and topiramate (TPM) (HR = 0.64; 95% CI 0.52–0.79).
- Adverse events were the most common reason for treatment failure in CBZ (102/177 = 58%), oxcarbazepine (OXA) (49/92 = 53%) and TPM (101/202 = 50%).
- Inadequate seizure control was the most common reason for treatment failure for GBP (99/209 = 47%).
- Inadequate seizure control (60/155 = 39%) and adverse events (39%) were both common reasons for treatment failure with LTG.

Criticisms and Limitations: This was an unblinded study. It did not include levetiracetam (LEV), zonisamide (ZNS), and pregabalin (PGP), which were licensed after the study started.[2] The major advantage of lamotrigine over carbamazepine in this study was tolerability. Questions were raised as to whether the study was biased against carbamazepine given titration to a higher than average efficacy dose of 400 mg in most adults with newly diagnosed epilepsy[3] and use of a less well-tolerated immediate-release formulation.[4]

Other Relevant Studies and Information:

- Many new anti-epileptic drugs are typically only compared to placebo in randomized clinical trials (RCTs) when seeking approval as add-on therapy.
- Prior to this study, the 2006 guidelines from the International League Against Epilepsy (ILAE) listed only CBZ and phenytoin (PHT) as adequate comparators for adults with partial-onset seizures.[5]
- Since 2006, in additional to this open-label RCT, there have been 2 new noninferiority trials comparing LEV and ZNS to controlled-release CBZ,[6,7] and other RCTs comparing TPM to PHT[8] and PGP to LTG.[9]
- Notably, a superiority RCT in 2005 comparing LTG and CBZ as a 24-week monotherapy found the seizure-free rate to be similar between 88 LTG and 88 CBZ patients.[10]
- The current 2013 ILAE recommendations for efficacious initial therapy for adults with partial-onset seizures, according to available trial data, are as follows:[11]
  - Established (level A): LEV, ZNS, CBZ, PHT

- Probably (level B): VPA
- Possibly (level C): GBP, LTG, OXC, phenobarbital, TPM, vigabatrin
- Potentially (level D): Clonazepam, primidone

Summary and Implications: For patients with partial seizures, lamotrigine (LTG) had the lowest rate of treatment failure compared to all drugs (CBZ, TPM, GBP). It did not reach statistical significance with oxcarbazepine, which had a smaller number of patients. The superiority of lamotrigine over carbamazepine was due to its better tolerability. While this study was only considered class III evidence by the ILAE given its open-label design and disqualified LTG for the level A rating for efficacy, it involved over 1,700 patients and completed close to 8,000 patient-years of follow-up, providing pragmatic guidance.

CLINICAL CASE: INITIAL TREATMENT OF NEWLY DIAGNOSED PARTIAL-ONSET EPILEPSY

Case History:

A 32-year-old man with a history of traumatic brain injury after a motor vehicle accident presents to your epilepsy outpatient office after he developed involuntary twitching that typically starts in his left thumb. In less than 1 minute, his typical seizure spreads to involve his entire left hand, forearm and face. He has no recollection of events afterwards, but has been told he usually falls down, with twitching involving his whole left hemibody. He has bitten his tongue and lost urinary continence. He has been unresponsive for up to 5 minutes and confused for up to an hour afterwards. He is a truck driver. His wife reports he has previously stopped various medications because of side effects.

MRI of the brain shows few small areas consistent with hemosiderin deposits on gradient echo sequences.

Based on the results of this trial, what treatment options would you consider for this patient?

Suggested Answer:

The patient in this vignette has symptoms consistent with partial-onset seizures with secondary generalization, presumably from a seizure focus from his prior TBI.

The SANAD trial demonstrated that fewer patients with partial seizures experienced treatment failure on lamotrigine versus carbamazepine (12% fewer at 1 year, 8% fewer at 2 years, overall HR = 0.78), mostly due to its better tolerability. Lamotrigine is not inferior to carbamazepine in time to treatment failure as defined by inadequate seizure control.

The most common clinically important adverse events reported in the trial for carbamazepine was tiredness, drowsiness, fatigue, and lethargy (36/378 per protocol for CBZ, 17/378 for LTG). There is hence evidence to support starting LTG as initial monotherapy for good efficacy and better tolerability. Alternately, controlled-release CBZ or the newer agents LEV or ZNS could also be considered, given level A recommendations by the latest ILAE guidelines. Expected side effects, the importance of seizure control, and implications for driving should be discussed with the patient.

References

1. Marson AG et al. The SANAD study of effectiveness of carbamazepine, gabapentin, lamotrigine, oxcarbazepine or topiramate for treatment of partial epilepsy: an unblended randomized controlled trial. *Lancet.* 2007;369(9566):1000–1015.
2. Panayiotopoulos CP. Old versus new antiepileptic drugs: the SANAD study. *Lancet.* 2007;370:313–314.
3. Brodie MJ et al. Comparison of levetiracetam and controlled-release carbamazepine in newly diagnosed epilepsy. *Neurology.* 2007;68:402–408.
4. Saetre E et al. An international multicenter randomized double-blind controlled trial of lamotrigine and sustained-release carbamazepine in the treatment of newly diagnosed epilepsy in the elderly. *Epilepsia.* 2007;48:1292–1302.
5. Glauser T et al. ILAE treatment guidelines: Evidence-based analysis of antiepileptic drug efficacy and effectiveness as initial monotherapy for epileptic seizures. *Epilepsia.* 2006;47(7):1094–1120.
6. Brodie MJ et al. Comparison of levetiracetam and controlled-release carbamazepine in newly diagnosed epilepsy. *Neurology.* 2007;68:402–408.
7. Baulac M et al. Comparison of the efficacy and tolerability of zonisamide and controlled release carbamazepine in the newly diagnosed partial epilepsy: a phase 3, randomized, double-blind, non-inferiority trial. *Lancet Neurol.* 2012;11:579–588.
8. Ramsay E et al. Efficacy, tolerability, and safety of rapidly initiation of topiramate versus phenytoin in patients with new-onset epilepsy: a randomized double-blind clinical trial. *Epilepsia.* 2010;51:1970–1977.
9. Kwan et al. Efficacy and safety of pregabalin versus lamotrigine in patients with newly diagnosed partial seizures: a phase 3, double-blind, randomized, parallel-group trial. *Lancet Neurol.* 2011;10:881–890.
10. Steinhoff BJ et al. The LAM-SAFE study: lamotrigine versus carbamazepine or valproic acid in newly diagnosed focal and generalized epilepsies in adolescents and adults. *Seizure.* 2005;14:597–605.
11. Glauser et al. Updated ILAE evidence review of antiepileptic drug efficacy and effectiveness as initial monotherapy for epileptic seizures and syndromes. *Epilepsia.* 2013;54(3):551–563.

5

Valproate for Generalized and Unclassifiable Epilepsy

Arm B of the SANAD Trial

SHIVANI GHOSHAL

> For patients with generalised onset seizures or seizures that are difficult to classify, valproate is significantly more effective than topiramate for treatment failure and significantly more effective than lamotrigine for 12-month remission. Thus valproate should remain a first-line treatment for such patients.
>
> —MARSON ET AL.[1]

Research Question: What are the relative efficacies and longer-term effects of valproate, lamotrigine, and topiramate for patients with generalized onset seizures or seizures that are difficult to classify?[1]

Funding: Funded by the Health Technology Assessment UK Programme, with an additional 20% of resources coming from companies with products assessed.

Year Study Began: 1999

Year Study Published: 2007

Study Location: Multicenter trial in the United Kingdom

Who Was Studied: Patients were referred if they (1) had a history of 2 or more clinically definite and unprovoked epileptic seizures in the preceding year and (2) the recruiting physician regarded valproate as a more appropriate standard of treatment than carbamazepine.

Who Was Excluded: Patients were excluded if they (1) were aged <4 years, (2) had acute symptomatic seizures (such as febrile seizures), and (3) had a history of progressive neurologic disease.

How Many Patients: 716

Study Overview: See Table 5.1 for the study design.

Table 5.1. STUDY DESIGN

Drug	Randomized Patients Allocated (N = 716)
Lamotrigine	239
Topiramate	239
Valproate	238

Study Intervention: After the initial choice of drug was randomized, clinicians decided subsequent changes in dose or preparation, to most accurately mirror everyday practice. Online guidelines were available for clinicians as needed.

Follow-Up: Mean follow-up time was 30 months.

Endpoints: Primary outcomes: Time to treatment failure (stopping the randomized drug because of inadequate seizure control, intolerable side effects, or both); the addition of other antiepileptic drugs; and time to 1-year remission of seizures. Secondary outcomes: Time from randomization to a first seizure; time to achieve a two-year remission; frequency of clinically important adverse events; and side effects.

RESULTS

- For time to treatment failure for any reason: Valproate is superior to topiramate, with lamotrigine intermediate. The effect is greater for patients with idiopathic generalized epilepsy (Table 5.2).

- For adequate seizure control: Lamotrigine was found to have almost twice the failure rate of valproate. Topiramate also appeared to have a higher failure rate than valproate, though the result was not statistically significant.
- Intention-to-treat analysis, per protocol, for 1-year remission: Valproate is more effective than lamotrigine and topiramate.
- For quality adjusted life-year (QALY) studies, topiramate and lamotrigine have positive incremental costs and negative incremental seizures—and were therefore both inferior to valproate.

Table 5.2. HAZARD RATIOS FOR LAMOTRIGINE AND TOPIRAMATE COMPARED TO VALPROATE

Endpoint	Lamotrigine	Topiramate
Time to treatment failure	HR 1.25 (95% CI 0.94–1.68)	HR 1.57 (95% CI 1.19–2.08)
Time to treatment failure for idiopathic generalized epilepsy	HR 1.55 (95% CI 1.07–2.24)	HR 1.89 (95% CI 1.32–2.70)
For inadequate seizure control	HR 1.95 (95% CI 1.28–2.98)	HR 1.45 (95% CI 0.92–2.27)
For 1-year remission (intention-to-treat analysis, per protocol)	HR 0.76 (95% CI 0.60–0.95)	HR 0.77 (95% CI 0.61–0.97)

Criticisms and Limitations: This study was unblinded and relied heavily on perceived time to treatment failure. However, SANAD also attempted to best mirror clinical practice and titration; a blinded study would be less representative of clinician practice. EEG and neuroimaging were optional for these patients; their diagnosis of seizure and epilepsy was based on clinical suspicion and it is possible that some study participants didn't have true epilepsy. The pooled population of patients in the sections of this study had a variety of different types of epilepsy, and it is difficult to know how each seizure type responded to the study medications. Levetiracetam is now frequently used as monotherapy for patients aged >16 years with unexplained seizures. The drug was unfortunately not addressed in this study, despite its popular use, as it was introduced to the market after the study's inception. Finally, there were more men than women in this study, likely influenced by the fact that valproate has known teratogenic effects and clinicians were reluctant to randomize women of child-bearing age to possible treatment with valproate.

Other Relevant Studies and Information:

- The 2013 ILAE (International League Against Epilepsy) guidelines now incorporate SANAD I findings for treatment of patients with generalized-onset seizures. Valproate is now considered first-line therapy for patients with generalized-onset or unclassifiable epilepsy.[2]
- In April 2013, SANAD II started as a comparison of effectiveness and quality of life between levetiracetam, zonisamide, and other standard treatments for epilepsy.
- Recent post-hoc subgroup analyses of data from the original SANAD trials further examined a variety of clinical factors for outcome prediction. Significant factors for 12-month remission included sex, treatment history, age, and total number of seizures prior to randomization.[3]

Summary and Implications: In comparison to lamotrigine and topiramate, valproate remains a superior treatment for time to treatment failure in patients with generalized seizures and idiopathic generalized epilepsy, and should remain a first-line therapy for these patients.[2]

CLINICAL CASE: AED SELECTION IN PATIENTS WITH IDIOPATHIC GENERALIZED EPILEPSY CURRENTLY ON VALPROATE THERAPY

Case History:
A 29-year old gentleman presents to your clinic after his second unprovoked seizure. He is otherwise healthy. Clinically he appears to have idiopathic generalized epilepsy. He had been started on valproate, though he is interested in "newer" anti-epileptic drugs—specifically, lamotrigine and topiramate. He wonders whether lamotrigine would be a better treatment for seizure control. Based on SANAD's findings, what would you counsel?

Suggested Answer:
Valproate is superior to both topiramate and lamotrigine for seizure control—especially in patients with idiopathic generalized epilepsy. The patient should continue on his current anti-epileptic therapy if he tolerates the medication well.

References

1. Marson AG, Al-Kharusi AM, et al. The SANAD study of effectiveness of valproate, lamotrigine, or topiramate for generalised and unclassifiable epilepsy: an unblinded randomized controlled trial. *Lancet Neurol.* 2007;369(3):1016–1026.
2. Glauser T, Ben-Menachem E, Bourgeois B, et al. Updated ILAE evidence review of antiepileptic drug efficacy and effectiveness as initial monotherapy for epileptic seizures and syndromes. *Epilepsia.* 2013;54(3):551–563.
3. Bonnett L, Smith CT, Smith D, et al. Time to 12-month remission and treatment failure for generalized and unclassified epilepsy. *J Neurol Neurosurg Psychiatr.* 2014; 85(6):603–610.

SECTION III

Headache

6

Sumatriptan for Acute Migraine

ALLISON ARCH

> We conclude that 6 mg of sumatriptan given subcutaneously is an effective, rapid, and well-tolerated acute treatment for migraine attacks.
> —The Subcutaneous Sumatriptan International Study Group[1]

Research Question: Is subcutaneous sumatriptan, a selective agonist of 5-$HT_{1B/D/F}$ receptors, effective as an abortive therapy for migraine attacks?[1]

Year Study Began: 1989

Year Published: 1991

Study Location: 58 hospital neurology departments, pain clinics, and physicians' offices in 10 countries.

Who Was Studied: Patients aged 18–65 years at the time of a migraine headache, as defined by the International Headache Society's Headache Classification Committee. All patients had a history of migraines for at least 1 year, and a maximum of 6 attacks per month.

Who Was Excluded: Patients with ischemic heart disease; peripheral vascular disease; renal, hepatic, or cardiac impairment; epilepsy; stroke;

blood pressure ≥160/95; serious psychiatric illness; and pregnant women. Headache patients who were reliant on opiates or other drugs were also excluded. Those who had taken prophylactic migraine medications within 2 weeks, ergot-containing preparations within 24 hours, or simple analgesic or nonsteroidal anti-inflammatory drugs within 6 hours were excluded as well.

How Many Patients: 639

Study Overview: See Figure 6.1 for a summary of the study design.

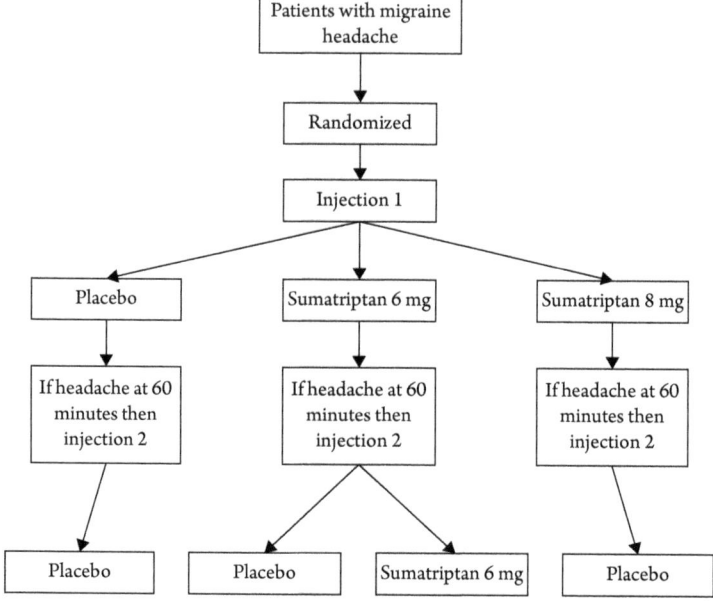

Figure 6.1 Summary of Subcutaneous Sumatriptan Study Design.

Study Intervention: Patients with acute migraine headache were randomized to receive subcutaneous sumatriptan 6 mg, 8 mg, or placebo. At 60 minutes if they still had a headache, subjects in the sumatriptan 8 mg and initial placebo groups all received a placebo injection. If patients initially received sumatriptan 6 mg and still had a headache at 60 minutes, they were randomized to either a second injection of sumatriptan 6 mg or to placebo.

Follow-Up: 30, 60, and 120 minutes, then 2–5 days.

Endpoints: Primary outcome: relief of headache from "severe or moderate" to "mild or none," 30, 60, and 120 minutes after the first injection. Secondary outcomes: pain freedom, need for usual rescue medications at 120 minutes; relief of nausea, vomiting, photophobia, phonophobia; functional disability; recurrence of headache within 24 hours after treatment; adverse events.

RESULTS

- The median duration of headache before initiation of treatment was 425 minutes in the 6 mg sumatriptan group, 421 minutes in the 8 mg group, and 357 minutes in the placebo group.
- As compared with the placebo group, 47% more patients who received 6 mg of sumatriptan and 54% more patients who received 8 mg of sumatriptan had improvement in severity of headache at 60 minutes (primary endpoint; $P < 0.001$).
- At 120 minutes, headache severity was improved in 75% of patients treated with 6 mg of sumatriptan plus placebo, 81% of patients treated with two 6 mg injections of sumatriptan, 82% of patients given 8 mg of sumatriptan plus placebo, and 30% of patients given two injections of placebo (see Table 6.1). The response rates of the three sumatriptan regimens did not differ significantly from each other, but all three were significantly better than the response rate in patients treated with placebo only ($P < 0.001$).
- Sumatriptan was significantly more effective than placebo in relieving nausea, vomiting, photophobia, and phonophobia.
- Treatment with sumatriptan markedly improved ability to function normally: at 60 minutes, 45% could function normally compared with 9% treated with placebo; at 120 minutes, the numbers were 78% versus 22%.
- Rescue medication was taken by 44% of those who received placebo alone, and 8%–12% of those assigned to any sumatriptan regimen.
- Proportion of headache recurrence within 24 hours was 34%–38% in sumatriptan-treated patients versus 18% in placebo.
- The most frequent adverse events in the sumatriptan group were injection site reaction, flushing, and a feeling of heaviness.

Table 6.1. RESPONSE RATES 120 MINUTES AFTER THE FIRST INJECTION

	Placebo + Placebo	6 mg Sumatriptan + Placebo	6 mg Sumatriptan + 6 mg Sumatriptan	8 mg Sumatriptan + Placebo
Total number of patients	92	110	106	49
Number with improvement (%)	28 (30%)	83 (75%)	86 (81%)	40 (82%)

Criticisms and Limitations: Many groups of patients were excluded from this study, including those recently on preventive therapies for migraine headaches. Patients with serious comorbidities were also excluded.

Other Relevant Studies:

- An additional randomized study of 136 patients with migraine found that 6 mg of subcutaneous sumatriptan was effective in treating acute migraine in the ED compared with placebo. In patients with headache recurrence within 24 hours, oral sumatriptan (100 mg) was effective as abortive therapy for the recurrence.[2]
- A randomized double-blind study examined the efficacy of a second subcutaneous dose of 6 mg sumatriptan in patients with headache recurrence. These patients had initially been successfully treated with 6 mg subcutaneous sumatriptan for a migraine attack. Fifteen percent of the study population had headache recurrence, and their recurrence was effectively treated by a further dose of subcutaneous sumatriptan.[3]
- The American Headache Society evidence-based guidelines on the assessment of migraine pharmacotherapies gives sumatriptan (oral, nasal spray, injectable, and the transcutaneous patch) level A evidence for its efficacy in treating acute migraine attacks.[4]

Summary and Implications: A single subcutaneous sumatriptan injection rapidly relieved the headache and other symptoms of a migraine attack. It was also well tolerated. Up to a third of responders, however, experienced headache recurrence within 24 hours. Later studies have shown that a recurring headache responds equally well to a repeated dose of sumatriptan. A second dose at 1 hour in patients who did not show initial response did not afford additional benefit. Most patients rated treatment with sumatriptan as good or excellent. It is an effective strategy for abortive treatment in migraine headaches.

CLINICAL CASE: ABORTIVE THERAPY FOR ACUTE MIGRAINE HEADACHE

Case History:
A 27-year-old woman with a history of migraine headaches presented to the emergency department with a bifrontal headache that started 3 hours prior. It was of similar quality but more severe than her typical headache. She had accompanying nausea, vomiting, and photophobia. Is subcutaneous sumatriptan an effective treatment strategy for this patient?

Suggested Answer:
This patient has few medical comorbidities and is a good candidate for sumatriptan therapy. According to the subcutaneous sumatriptan randomized clinical trial, 6 mg of subcutaneous sumatriptan likely will be effective at reducing the severity of her headache and its accompanying symptoms within 1 hour. The medication is well tolerated. Around 35% of patients will experience headache recurrence within the next 24 hours, however. The patient should be counseled that this may occur and that a repeated dose of sumatriptan likely will treat the headache recurrence effectively.

References

1. Treatment of migraine attacks with sumatriptan—The Subcutaneous Sumatriptan International Study Group. *N Engl J Med*. 1991;325(5):316–321.
2. Akpunonu BE, Mutgi AB, Federman DJ, et al. Subcutaneous sumatriptan for treatment of acute migraine in patients admitted to the emergency department: a multicenter study. *Ann Emerg Med*. 1995;25(4):464–469.
3. Cull RE, Price WH, Dunbar A. The efficacy of subcutaneous sumatriptan in the treatment of recurrence of migraine headache. *J Neurol Neurosurg Psychiatry*. 1997;62(5):490–495.
4. Marmura MJ, Silberstein SD, Schwedt TJ. The acute treatment of migraine in adults: the American Headache Society evidence assessment of migraine pharmacotherapies. *Headache*. 2015;55(1):3–20.

SECTION IV

Neuroinfectious Disease

7
Steroids for Bell's Palsy

BENJAMIN N. BLOND

> Our study showed that the administration of prednisolone can increase the probability of complete recovery (from facial nerve paralysis in Bell's palsy) at 9 months... Acyclovir produced no benefit over placebo...
> —SULLIVAN ET AL.[1]

Research Question: Does early therapy with prednisolone or acyclovir improve complete recovery from Bell's palsy?[1]

Funding: Health Technology Assessment Programme of the National Institute for Health Research (Department of Health, England).

Year Study Began: 2004

Year Study Published: 2007

Study Location: Multiple sites, mainly family practices, referring to 17 hospitals throughout Scotland.

Who Was Studied: Patients aged ≥16 years with unilateral facial nerve weakness with no identifiable cause who could be referred to a collaborating otorhinolaryngologist within 72 hours of symptom onset.

Who Was Excluded: Patients with any of the following conditions: pregnancy, breastfeeding, uncontrolled diabetes (HbA1c > 8%), peptic ulcer disease, suppurative otitis media, herpes zoster, multiple sclerosis, systemic infection, sarcoidosis and other rare conditions, and an inability to provide informed consent.

How Many Patients: 551

Study Overview: See Figure 7.1 for a summary of the study design.

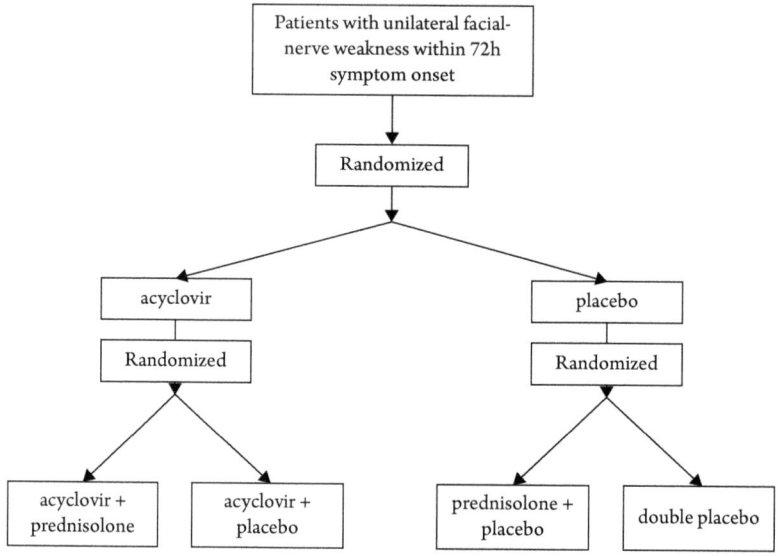

Figure 7.1 Summary of Study Design.

Study Intervention: Prednisolone, 25 mg twice daily, plus placebo (n = 138); acyclovir, 400 mg 5 times daily, plus placebo (n = 138); prednisolone plus acyclovir (n = 134); or both placebos (n = 141). Study drugs were taken for 10 days.

Follow-Up: Up to 9 months.

Endpoints: Primary outcome: facial nerve function as assessed by the House-Brackmann grading system (Table 7.1).[2] Secondary outcomes: health-related quality of life (Health Utilities Index Mark 3), facial appearance (Derriford Appearance Scale 59), and pain (Brief Pain Inventory).

Table 7.1. HOUSE-BRACKMANN FACIAL NERVE GRADING SYSTEM[a]

I	Normal and symmetric throughout
II	Slight weakness only noticeable with close inspection
	Can close eyes completely with minimal effort
	Slight asymmetry of full smile
	Synkinesis barely noticeable; contracture and/or spasm are absent
III	Obvious weakness, but not disfiguring appearance
	May or may not be able to lift eyebrow
	With maximal effort, can completely close eyes, and can make strong, albeit asymmetric movements of mouth
	Obvious, but not disfiguring synkinesis, mass movement, or spasm
IV	Obvious disfiguring weakness
	Unable to lift brow
	Unable to completely close and asymmetry of mouth despite maximal effort
	Severe synkinesis, mass movement, spasm
V	Motion barely perceptible on paretic side
	Incomplete eye closure, slight movement corner mouth
	Synkinesis, contracture, and spasm are usually absent
VI	No movement, loss of tone, no synkinesis, contracture, or spasm

[a] House JW, Brackmann DE. Facial nerve grading system. *Otolaryngol—Head Neck Surg.* 1985;93:146–147.

RESULTS

- 53.8% of patients initiated treatment within 24 hours, 32.1% within 48 hours, and 14.1% within 72 hours.
- For patients receiving double placebo, 64.7% were fully recovered after 3 months, and 85.2% after 9 months.
- At 3 months and 9 months, rates of complete recovery were higher with prednisolone versus placebo (see Tables 7.2). At 3 months, the absolute risk reduction was 19%, and the number needed to treat to achieve one additional complete recovery was 6. At 9 months, the absolute risk reduction was 12% and the number needed to treat was 8.
- There was no significant difference between the complete recovery rates in the acyclovir comparison groups at 3 or 9 months (see Tables 7.2 & 7.3).
- There were no significant differences among the study groups in secondary measures of health-related quality of life, facial appearance, and pain, except the quality of life at 9 months was significantly higher ($P = 0.04$) in patients who did not receive prednisolone. However, given that secondary measures were obtained only in patients who had not recovered in 3 months, and given the multiple comparisons, this result should be interpreted with caution.

Table 7.2. SUMMARY OF KEY FINDINGS—PREDNISOLONE

Outcome	Prednisolone	No Prednisolone	P value
% Complete facial nerve recovery (House-Brackmann I) at 3 months	83.0%	63.6%	<0.001
% Complete facial nerve recovery (House-Brackmann I) at 9 months	94.4%	81.6%	<0.001

Table 7.3. SUMMARY OF KEY FINDINGS—ACYCLOVIR

Outcome	Acyclovir	No Acyclovir	P value
% Complete facial nerve recovery (House-Brackmann I) at 3 months	71.2%	75.7%	0.5
% Complete facial nerve recovery (House-Brackmann I) at 9 months	85.4%	90.8%	0.1

Criticisms and Limitations: This was an exclusively Scottish patient population and the results may not apply to other populations. The House-Brackmann scale lacks sensitivity to change in facial function compared to other, more arduous scales, such as the Sydney and Sunnybrook grading systems. Additionally, the dose of antiviral therapy was questioned as potentially insufficient to produce a benefit.

Other Relevant Studies and Information:

- An additional large randomized double-blind placebo-controlled trial by Engström et al. confirmed the benefits of prednisolone, demonstrating increased rates of complete recovery of facial nerve paralysis at 3, 6, and 12 months, as well as decreased times to recovery.[3]
- Based on these studies, the AAN highly recommends offering steroids in new onset Bell's palsy to increase the probability of recovery of facial nerve function (2 class I studies, level A).[4]
- The use of antiviral therapy remains controversial. Several studies have suggested a possible benefit of the addition of antiviral therapy, at least in subgroups with severe facial nerve palsy.[5,6] However, these studies were smaller or suffered from methodological limitations, such as a lack of appropriate double blinding. Other studies have failed to demonstrate a benefit of antiviral therapy.[3,7,8] This includes the study by Engström et al., which is the largest trial and is a randomized double-blind placebo-controlled study. Engström et al. tested valacyclovir, which has higher bioavailability than acyclovir, but failed to find a benefit of antiviral therapy. Given that a small benefit

of antiviral therapy has not been excluded, professional organizations recommend that adding antiviral therapy could be considered in the appropriate clinical situations, but this would be based on lower-quality evidence and would be expected to only be of modest benefit.[4]

Summary and Implications: The study by Sullivan et al. demonstrates that corticosteroid therapy within 72 hours of symptom onset is effective in increasing the rate of complete recovery of facial nerve function at 3 and 9 months in Bell's palsy in a large double-blind placebo-controlled trial. However, the study did not demonstrate more rapid recovery with acyclovir treatment compared to placebo, casting doubt on the benefit of antiviral therapy in Bell's palsy.

CLINICAL CASE: TREATMENT OF BELL'S PALSY

Case History:
A 40-year-old gentleman presents to your office 24 hours after the initial onset of facial paralysis. He states that he suddenly noticed he could not move the left side of his face. He also thinks that his sense of taste may be impaired, and that sounds appear louder to him in his left ear. After performing a history and physical and ensuring that the patient has a peripheral seventh nerve palsy, you believe the most likely diagnosis is Bell's palsy. The patient is very concerned about his face and asks if there is anything you can do to improve his condition. Based on the results of Sullivan et al., how would you treat the patient?

Suggested Answer:
Bell's palsy is an idiopathic condition with possible viral and autoimmune etiologies. Sullivan et al. demonstrated the benefits of corticosteroid therapy within 72 hours of symptom onset in increasing the rate of complete recovery. The patient does not have any significant contraindications to corticosteroid therapy, such as poorly controlled diabetes, and so he should be started on prednisolone 25 mg twice daily, or an equivalent dosing of another corticosteroid. Eye protection should be provided if the patient has impaired eye closure. Additional testing for alternate causes of facial nerve palsies, such as Lyme disease, HIV, Ramsay-Hunt syndrome, zoster sine herpetica, sarcoidosis, multiple sclerosis, and parotid tumors should be performed as clinically indicated by a careful history and physical exam, as these conditions require different treatment. In the absence of specific viral diagnoses, such as herpes zoster reactivation, the addition of antiviral therapy for the treatment of facial nerve palsy remains considerably more controversial. The preponderance of

evidence seems to favor the findings of Sullivan et al., that the addition of antiviral therapy does not increase the rate of facial nerve recovery. However, a modest effect has not been entirely excluded, and physicians may consider adding antiviral therapy in certain clinical situations. Overall, the patient can be reassured about the good prognosis of his condition based on the high percentage of patients with complete recovery of facial nerve function after prednisolone treatment.

References

1. Sullivan FM, Swan IRC, Donnan PT, et al. Early treatment with prednisolone or acyclovir in Bell's palsy. *N Engl J Med.* 2007;357:1598–1607.
2. House, JW, Brackmann, DE. Facial nerve grading system. *Otolaryngol—Head Neck Surg.* 1985;93:146–147.
3. Engström M, Berg T, Stjemquist-Desatnik A, et al. Prednisolone and valacyclovir in Bell's palsy: a randomised double-blind, placebo controlled, multicentre trial. *Lancet Neurol.* 2008;7:993–1000.
4. Gronseth GS, Paduga R. Evidence-based guideline update: steroids and antivirals for Bell palsy: report of the Guideline Development Subcommittee of the American Academy of Neurology. *Neurology.* 2012;79(22):2209–2213.
5. Hato N, Yamada H, Kohno H, et al. Valacyclovir and prednisolone treatment for Bell's palsy: a multicenter, randomized, placebo-controlled study. *Otol Neurotol.* 2007;28:408–413.
6. Minnerop M, Herbst M, Fimmers R, Matz B, Klockgether T, Wullner U. Bell's palsy: combined treatment of famciclovir and prednisone is superior to prednisone alone. *J Neurol.* 2008;255:1726–1730.
7. Kawaguchi K, Inamura H, Abe Y, et al. Reactivation of herpes simplex virus type 1 and varicella-zoster virus and therapeutic effects of combination therapy with prednisolone and valacyclovir in patients with Bell's palsy. *Laryngoscope.* 2007;117:147–156.
8. Yeo SG, Lee YC, Park DC, Cha CI. Acyclovir and steroid versus steroid alone in the treatment of Bell's palsy. *Am J Otolaryngol.* 2008;29:163–168.

8

Steroids for Acute Bacterial Meningitis

ROBERT J. CLAYCOMB

> Early treatment with dexamethasone improves the outcome in adults with acute bacterial meningitis....
>
> —DE GANS ET AL.[1]

Research Question: Do intravenous corticosteroids in combination with appropriate antibiotic therapies improve neurological outcomes in adults with likely bacterial meningitis?[1]

Funding: Supported in part by NV Organon (a pharmaceutical company in the Netherlands, now part of Merck).

Year Study Began: 1993

Year Study Published: 2002

Study Location: 50 sites within the Netherlands, Belgium, Germany, Denmark, and Austria.

Who Was Studied: Patients aged ≥17 years, who had suspected meningitis, and who had (1) cloudy cerebrospinal fluid, (2) cerebrospinal fluid with bacteria present on Gram stain, or (3) pleocytosis >1,000 cells/mm³.

Who Was Excluded: Patients with (1) previous hypersensitivity reaction to either β-lactam antibiotics or corticosteroids, (2) pregnancy, (3) a cerebrospinal shunt, (4) antibiotic treatment within the previous 48 hours, (5) an active fungal or tuberculosis infection, (6) recent head trauma, (7) a recent neurosurgical procedure, (8) peptic ulcer disease, or (9) participation in another clinical trial.

How Many Patients: 301

Study Overview: See Figure 8.1 for a summary of the study design.

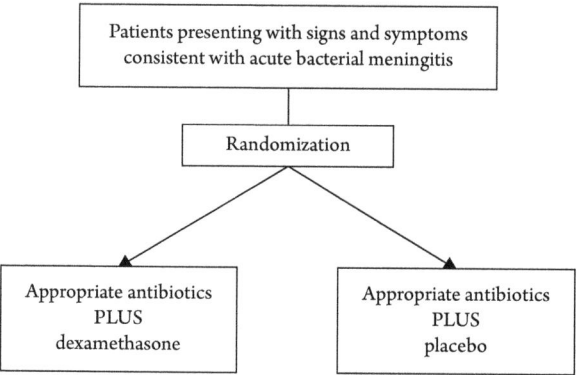

Figure 8.1 Summary of Study Design.

Study Intervention: Patients randomized to receive adjunctive corticosteroids in addition to appropriate antibiotics received dexamethasone 10 mg IV every 6 hours for 4 days. Patients randomized to receive placebo received an identical-appearing IV placebo every 6 hours for 4 days. Either the dexamethasone or the placebo was given within 20 minutes of antibiotic therapy. The antibiotic therapy initially consisted of ampicillin, but the study protocol was modified after the trial began so that empiric therapy could be consistent with local protocols. Subsequent treatment was further tailored to the Gram stain and culture results.

Follow-Up: 8 weeks.

Endpoints: Primary outcome of disability was determined by Glasgow Outcome Scale score (GOS, see Table 8.1).[2] GOS were also dichotomized into favorable outcomes (scores of 5) and unfavorable outcomes (scores 1–4). Secondary outcomes measures included (1) death, (2) focal neurological deficit (aphasia, cranial nerve deficit, monoparesis, hemiparesis, and severe ataxia), (3) hearing loss, (4) gastrointestinal bleeding, (5) fungal infection, (6) herpes zoster infection, and (7) hyperglycemia (>144 mg/dL).

Table 8.1. GLASGOW OUTCOME SCALE

Score	Description
1	Death
2	A vegetative state, patient unable to interact with environment
3	Severe disability, patient unable to live independently but can follow commands
4	Moderate disability, patient can live independently but unable to return to school or work
5	Mild or no disability

Adapted from Jennett et al. Assessment of outcome after severe brain damage. *Lancet.* 1975;1(7905):480–484.

RESULTS

- Dexamethasone led to better outcomes than placebo, particularly among patients with meningitis due to *Streptococcus pneumoniae* (see Tables 8.2 and 8.3).
- Patients who presented with an initial clinical exam consistent with a Glasgow Coma Scale of 8–11 appeared to have the greatest benefit of adjunctive dexamethasone.
- There was no statistically significant difference in the incidence of gastrointestinal bleeding, hyperglycemia, fungal infections, or herpes zoster infections between dexamethasone- and placebo-treated patients.

Table 8.2. SUMMARY OF KEY FINDINGS

Outcome	Dexamethasone Group (n = 157)	Placebo Group (n = 144)	P Value
Unfavorable Outcome	15%	25%	0.03
Mortality	7%	15%	0.04
Focal Neurological Deficit	13%	20%	0.13
Hearing Loss	9%	12%	0.54

Table 8.3. Subgroup Analysis of Unfavorable Outcome by Isolated Pathogen

Unfavorable Outcome	Dexamethasone Group (n = 157)	Placebo Group (n = 144)	P Value
All pathogens	15%	25%	0.03
Streptococcus pneumoniae	26%	52%	0.006
Neisseria meningitidis	8%	11%	0.74
Other bacteria	17%	6%	0.55
Negative bacterial culture	0%	7%	0.40

Criticisms and Limitations: The study found a decrease in unfavorable outcomes and death, particularly among those with acute bacterial meningitis due to *S. pneumoniae*; however, the study was inadequately powered to detect significant benefits for other causative organisms. Dexamethasone is also thought to decrease blood–brain permeability, and its effect on the penetration of vancomycin in particular into the subarachnoid space remains a concern, especially in locations with higher rates of antibiotic resistance where vancomycin may be the most effective medication.

Other Relevant Studies and Information:

- Previous *in vivo* animal models of acute bacterial meningitis demonstrated that inflammation within the subarachnoid space, resulting from bacterial lysis, may contribute to poor outcomes.[3,4] This suggested that anti-inflammatory therapies may improve outcomes. Moreover, previous studies examining the effect of corticosteroids in pediatric populations demonstrated improved neurological outcomes.[5]
- A recent meta-analysis that examined 25 studies and over 4,000 patients confirmed the results of de Gans et al.[1] and demonstrated that adjunctive corticosteroids decrease poor neurological outcomes but do not necessarily reduce overall mortality.[6] However, a subgroup analysis did reveal that corticosteroids did decrease mortality in those patients with acute bacterial meningitis due to *S. pneumoniae*. Interestingly, the beneficial effects of corticosteroids were only seen in high-income countries.[6]
- The most recent treatment guidelines from the Infectious Diseases Society of America also recommend adjuvant corticosteroids for adults with suspected or proven pneumococcal meningitis.[7]

Summary and Implications: This study demonstrated that adjunctive dexamethasone therapy is associated with improved neurological outcomes for patients with likely bacterial meningitis, particularly S. *pneumoniae*, and is not associated with any clinically significant adverse events.

CLINICAL CASE: DEXAMETHASONE FOR ACUTE BACTERIAL MENINGITIS

Case History:
A 45-year-old man with a history of type 2 diabetes, hypertension, and gastroesophageal reflux disease (GERD) developed a severe holocephalic headache over the course of 1 day that was associated with moderate neck stiffness, nausea, vomiting, and subjective fever. He planned on visiting his primary care physician in the next few days; however, his headache worsened and he developed left hemiparesis. He was then brought to the emergency department for emergent evaluation.

On examination, he was tachycardic, normotensive and febrile to 102.5°F. He was profoundly encephalopathic and had a moderate left hemiparesis. His Glasgow Coma Score was 9. A rapid CT scan of the head demonstrated no acute intracranial process, and a lumbar puncture was performed. Opening pressure was elevated to 38 cm of H_2O and the fluid appeared cloudy. Gram stain revealed numerous Gram-positive cocci in chains, a glucose of 25 mg/dL, and a protein of 207 mg/dL. Cell counts revealed a pleocytosis of 1,125 cells/mm^3, 87% of which were neutrophils.

Within 45 minutes of arrival to the emergency department, IV antibiotics were started.

Should this patient be treated with adjunctive corticosteroids?

Suggested Answer:
Yes. This patient has acute bacterial meningitis and the likely causative organism is *S. pneumoniae*. Despite having preexisting comorbidities that may be exacerbated by corticosteroid use (type 2 diabetes and GERD), given his poor initial exam, he would likely benefit from adjunctive dexamethasone therapy.

References

1. de Gans J et al. Dexamethasone in adults with bacterial meningitis. *N Engl J Med*. 2002;347(20):1549–1556.
2. Jennett B, Bond M. Assessment of outcome after severe brain damage. *Lancet*. 1975;1(7905):480–484.

3. Täuber MG, Khayam-Bashi H, Sande MA. Effects of ampicillin and corticosteroids on brain water content, cerebrospinal fluid pressure, and cerebrospinal fluid lactate levels in experimental pneumococcal meningitis. *J Infect Dis.* 1985;151(3):528–534.
4. Scheld WM, Dacey RG, Winn HR, et al. Cerebrospinal fluid outflow resistance in rabbits with experimental meningitis. Alterations with penicillin and methylprednisolone. *J Clin Invest.* 1980;66(2):243–253.
5. McIntyre PB, Berkey CS, King SM, et al. Dexamethasone as adjunctive therapy in bacterial meningitis. A meta-analysis of randomized clinical trials since 1988. *JAMA.* 1997;278(11):925–931.
6. Brouwer MC, McIntyre P, Prasad K, van de Beek D. Corticosteroids for acute bacterial meningitis. *Cochrane Database Syst Rev.* 2013;6:CD004405.
7. Tunkel AR, Hartman BJ, Kaplan SL, et al. Practice guidelines for the management of bacterial meningitis. *Clin Infect Dis.* 2004;39(9):1267–1284.

SECTION V

Movement Disorders

9

Levodopa for Parkinson's Disease

SARAH E. BUCKINGHAM

> *The clinical data suggest that levodopa either slows progression of Parkinson's disease or has a prolonged effect on the symptoms of the disease.*
> —THE PARKINSON STUDY GROUP[1]

Research Question: Levodopa helps with symptoms of Parkinson's disease, but does it affect the course of Parkinson's disease?[1]

Funding: National Institute of Neurologic Disorders and Stroke, Department of Defense, General Clinical Research Center of the National Center for Research Resources, National Institutes of Health, and Teva Pharmaceuticals.

Year Study Began: 1998

Year Study Published: 2004

Study Location: 33 sites in the United States and 5 sites in Canada.

Who Was Studied: Patients aged ≥30 years who had received a diagnosis of Parkinson's disease within the past 2 years, had a rating < stage 3 on the modified Hoehn and Yahr Scale, and were considered not likely to require therapy for symptoms of the disease within the 9 months after enrollment in the study.

Modified Hoehn and Yahr Scale[2]
1.0: Unilateral involvement only
1.5: Unilateral and axial involvement
2.0: Bilateral involvement without impairment of balance
2.5: Mild bilateral disease with recovery on pull test
3.0: Mild to moderate bilateral disease; some postural instability; physically independent
4.0: Severe disability; still able to walk or stand unassisted
5.0: Wheelchair bound or bedridden unless aided

Who Was Excluded: Patients who were receiving antiparkinson medication, had been exposed to levodopa or to any dopamine agonist for >14 days, had an identifiable cause of parkinsonism, had a tremor in any limb that scored ≥3 on the Unified Parkinson's Disease Rating Scale (UPDRS), or had freezing of gait, loss of postural reflexes, major depression, or dementia.

How Many Patients: 361

Study Overview: See Figure 9.1 for a summary of the study design.

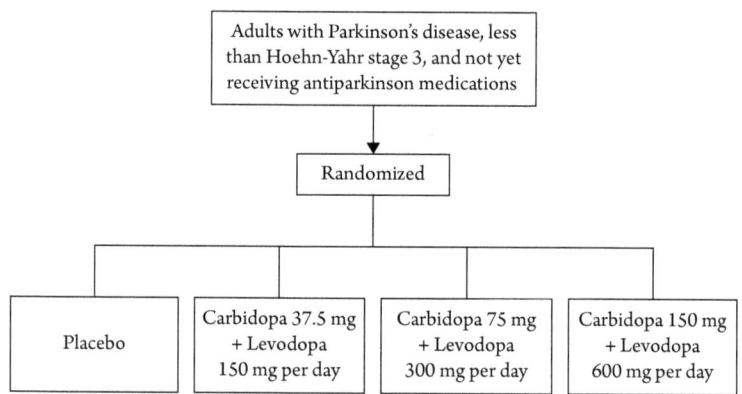

Figure 9.1 Summary of the Trial's Design.

Study Intervention: Patients were randomized to receive placebo or carbidopa-levodopa at a dose of 12.5/50 mg three times daily, 25/100 mg three times daily, or 50/200 mg three times daily, respectively. Additional antiparkinson medication was prohibited during the study period.

Follow-Up: 42 weeks.

Endpoints: Primary outcome: change in the severity of parkinsonism between the baseline visit and week 42, as measured by the total score on the UPDRS. Secondary outcome: change in the total scores on the UPDRS at each visit (weeks 3, 9, 24, and 40). Substudy: percentage change in the ratio of the specific striatal $[^{123}I]\beta$-CIT uptake to the nondisplaceable striatal $[^{123}I]\beta$-CIT uptake between SPECT imaging prior to baseline visit and at week 40.

The UPDRS is a commonly used scoring system to evaluate for cognitive, motor, and functional deficits. The first two sections are based on patients' responses, and the remainder is objectively evaluated by clinicians. The scale can be followed over time to assess progression of disease. A score of 0 represents no disability, whereas a score of 199 represents maximal disability. Below is a sample item on the UPDRS:

- Tremor at rest (head, upper, and lower extremities)
  0 = Absent
  1 = Slight and infrequently present
  2 = Mild in amplitude and persistent. Or moderate in amplitude, but only intermittently present.
  3 = Moderate in amplitude and present most of the time.
  4 = Marked in amplitude and present most of the time.

RESULTS

- Levodopa significantly reduced the worsening of symptoms of Parkinson's disease on the UPDRS at between baseline and the week 42 follow-up (see Table 9.1).
- The scores on the UPDRS in the three levodopa groups worsened during the 2-week washout period, but these groups did not deteriorate to the level observed in the placebo group. The group receiving the highest dose of levodopa had the best results.
- The total score on the UPDRS (means ± SD) showed a significant trend toward the reduction of symptoms with higher doses of levodopa. The effects of all three doses of levodopa differed significantly from the effect of the placebo. Scores on the UPDRS showed that treatment effects were significant for activities of daily living (ADL) and the motor component but not for the mental component.
- The adverse events that were significantly more common among those receiving levodopa at 600 mg daily than in placebo group were dyskinesias, nausea, infection, hypertonia, and headache (see Table 9.2).

- "The percent decrease (means ± SD) in striatal [^{123}I]β-CIT uptake over the 40 weeks of the study treatment was greater among subjects in the levodopa groups than in the placebo group, but this difference was not statistically significant."[1]
- "21 of the 142 subjects (14.7 percent) had a putaminal [^{123}I]β-CIT uptake of more than 3.25 at baseline."[1] SPECT analysis at week 40 excluding the 19 subjects without any dopaminergic deficit at baseline showed a significantly greater decrease in [^{123}I]β-CIT uptake among those receiving levodopa than among those receiving placebo.

Table 9.1. SUMMARY OF THE PRIMARY OUTCOME RESULTS: CHANGE IN UPDRS SCORE BETWEEN BASELINE AND WEEK 42 (AFTER THE WASHOUT PERIOD)

UPDRS Score	Placebo	Levodopa (mg/day)			P Value
		150	300	600	
Total score	7.8 ± 9.0	1.9 ± 6.0	1.9 ± 6.9	−1.4 ± 7.7	<0.001
Mental	0.3 ± 1.5	0.0 ± 1.5	0.1 ± 1.2	0.1 ± 1.4	0.18
ADL[a]	2.3 ± 3.4	0.5 ± 2.3	0.4 ± 2.9	−0.3 ± 3.0	<0.001
Motor	5.2 ± 6.4	1.4 ± 5.5	1.4 ± 5.3	−1.4 ± 5.9	<0.001

[a] Activities of daily living.

Table 9.2. SUMMARY OF THE IMAGING SUBSTUDY FINDINGS

Variable	Placebo	Levodopa (mg/day)			P Value for Dose-Response
		150	300	600	
Substudy Cohort					
Change (%)	−2.6 ± 11.3	−4.7 ± 10.8	−3.7 ± 9.1	−6.9 ± 8.1	0.15
P Value for comparison with placebo		0.46	0.63	0.11	
After exclusion of subjects with no dopaminergic deficit at baseline					
Change (%)	−1.4 ± 10.0	−6.0 ± 10.3	−4.0 ± 9.4	−7.2 ± 7.6	0.0036
P Value for comparison with placebo		0.16	0.40	0.015	

Criticisms and Limitations: Prior studies have suggested that a washout period of 32 days (4 half-lives) may be required to eliminate 90 percent of the drug's effects on symptoms; however in this study, a 2-week washout period was chosen. Following a full washout period, it is possible the benefit of the medication would be diminished or gone. In this study, there was a reduction in the worsening of symptoms based on UPDRS scores at baseline and week 42, compared to placebo, implying that symptom reduction remained despite withdrawal of study drug. As a subgroup analysis, 38 patients underwent a 4-week washout period, and there was no further worsening of the UPDRS scores during the additional 2 weeks.

Other Relevant Studies and Information:

- Other studies have investigated the effect of levodopa on dopamine-transporter binding with the use of neuroimaging. One study found a reduction in dopamine-transporter binding,[3] and others found no change in binding.[4-6] The sample sizes were too small in these studies to demonstrate statistical signifance.
- In vivo rodent studies suggest that levodopa can promote survival and enhance sprouting of nigral dopamine neurons.[7,8] The current study suggests that levodopa may slow progression of Parkinson's disease in humans.
- An open-label randomized trial by the PD MED Collaborative Group in the United Kingdom demonstrated long-term superiority of levodopa compared to levodopa-sparing agents regarding mobility, ADL, and overall quality of life.[9] During the 7-year follow-up period, the authors did not observe any deterioration of the clinical benefits of levodopa, suggesting that levodopa does not increase the progression of disease.
- The current guidelines, "Practice Parameter: Initiation of Treatment for Parkinson's Disease: An Evidence-Based Review," were published by the American Academy of Neurology in 2002 and reaffirmed in 2005. They are compatible with some aspects of this study and state, "Levodopa is more effective than cabergoline, ropinirole, and pramipexole in treating the motor and ADL features of PD."[10] The guidelines do not comment on the impact of medication on the progression of disease.

Summary and Implications: Levodopa, which is used to manage the symptoms of Parkinson's disease, did not increase the progression of disease. In fact, levodopa may slow disease progression, although the washout period in this study may have been inadequate for definitive evaluation. Small doses of levodopa were found to be effective, although less so than higher doses. High doses, however, were associated with a greater frequency of adverse events such as dyskinesia.

CLINICAL CASE: LEVODOPA FOR RECENTLY DIAGNOSED PARKINSON'S DISEASE

Case History:
A 61-year-old male presents with complaints of new-onset tremor and stiffness in his right hand. The tremor is mainly present at rest, and the stiffness in his right arm interferes with playing piano. His wife has noticed that he takes short, shuffling steps while walking. She also states that he overall moves more slowly than he did a few years ago.

On examination, he has a pill-rolling tremor at rest in his right hand, with cogwheel rigidity of his right upper extremity. Rapid alternating movements are slowed in the right upper and lower extremities. On gait examination, he has stooped posture, decreased arm swing on the right, short stride length, and shuffling steps. He demonstrates retropulsion on the pull test.

Clinically, he meets criteria for the diagnosis of Parkinson's disease. A workup for Parkinson's disease mimickers is negative. Based on the results of this study, should you treat this patient with levodopa?

Suggested Answer:
This study established that treatment with levodopa of patients with early Parkinson disease reduces symptoms and may slow the progression of disease. The patient in this vignette likely has early Parkinson's disease and would benefit from dopamine-replacing therapy for symptom management. Carbidopa-levodopa is a reasonable first choice and should be initiated at the lowest effective dose. This study showed that adverse events are more likely to occur with levodopa doses of 600 mg daily, and include dyskinesia, nausea, hypertonia, and headache. Newer data demonstrate that maintaining a levodopa dose of 400 mg daily or less reduces the risk of motor complications in particular.[11] A UPDRS evaluation may be completed at the initial visit prior to initiation of levodopa. This scale can be tracked over time to monitor progression of disease and response to therapy.

References

1. The Parkinson Study Group. Levodopa and the progression of Parkinson's disease. *N Engl J Med*. 2004;351:2498–2508.
2. Goetz CG, Poewe W, Rasol O, et al. Movement Disorder Society Task Force Report on the Hoehn and Yahr Staging Scale: status and recommendations. *Mov Disord*. 2004;19(9):1020–1028.
3. Guttman M, Stewart D, Hussey D, Wilson A, Houle S, Kish S. Influence of L-dopa and pramipexole on striatal dopamine transporter in early PD. *Neurology* 2001;56:1559–1564.

4. Parkinson Study Group. Dopamine transporter brain imaging to assess the effects of pramipexole vs levodopa on Parkinson disease progression. *JAMA.* 2002;287:1653–61.
5. Innis RB, Marek KL, Sheff K, et al. Effect of treatment with L-dopa/carbidopa or L-selegiline on striatal dopamine transporter SPECT imaging with [^{123}I]beta-CIT. *Mov Disord.* 1999;14:436–442.
6. Nurmi E, Bergman KJ, Eskola O, et al. Reproducibility and effect of levodopa on dopamine transporter function measurements: a [F-18]CFT PET study. *J Cereb Blood Flow Metab.* 2000;20:1604–1609.
7. Murer MG, Dziewczapolski G, Menalled LB, et al. Chronic levodopa is not toxic for remaining dopamine neurons, but instead promotes their recovery, in rats with moderate nigrostriatal lesions. *Ann Neurol.* 1998;43:561–575.
8. Datla KP, Blunt SB, Dexter DT. Chronic L-DOPA administration is not toxic to the remaining dopaminergic nigrostriatal neurons, but instead may promote their functional recovery, in rats with partial 6-OHDA or FeCl (3) nigrostriatal lesions. *Mov Disord.* 2001;16:424–434.
9. PD MED Collaborative Group. Long-term effectiveness of dopamine agonists and monoamine oxidase B inhibitors compared with levodopa as initial treatment for Parkinson's disease (PD MED): a large, open-label, pragmatic randomised trial. *Lancet.* 2014;384:1196–1205.
10. Miyasaki JM, Martin W, Suchowersky O, et al. Practice parameter: initiation of treatment for Parkinson's disease: an evidence-based review. *Neurology* 2002;58:11–17.
11. Stocchi F, Rascol O, Kieburtz K, et al. Initiating levodopa/carbidopa therapy with and without entacapone in early Parkinson disease: The STRIDE-PD study. *Ann Neurol.* 2010;68:18–27.

10

Deep-Brain Stimulation for Parkinson's Disease

SARAH E. BUCKINGHAM

This trial demonstrated the superior efficacy of neurostimulation over best medical management in patients with advanced Parkinson's disease and levodopa-related motor complications.
—Deuschl et al.[1]

Research Question: Is neurostimulation superior to best medical management in patients with advanced Parkinson's disease?[1]

Funding: German Federal Ministry of Education and Research.

Year Study Began: 2001

Year Study Published: 2006

Study Location: 10 academic centers in Germany and Austria.

Who Was Studied: Patients <75 years of age who received a clinical diagnosis of idiopathic Parkinson's disease at least 5 years previously and had parkinsonian motor symptoms or dyskinesias that limited their ability to perform activities of daily living (ADL), despite receiving optimal medical therapy.

Who Was Excluded: Patients with age ≥75 years, dementia, depression or psychosis, or contraindications to surgery.

How Many Patients: 156

Study Overview: See Figure 10.1 for a summary of the trial's design.

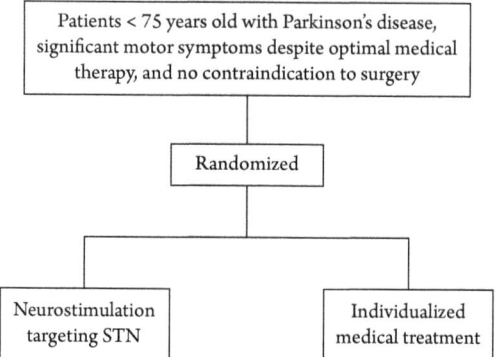

Figure 10.1 Summary of the Trial's Design.

Study Intervention: Patients were randomly assigned to neurostimulation or to best medical treatment. Patients assigned to the neurostimulation arm underwent bilateral stereotactic surgery under local anesthesia, targeting the subthalamic nucleus. The final implantation point of the microelectrode was the position at which the most significant effect on rigidity and other symptoms of Parkinson's disease was obtained, at the lowest stimulation intensity and with the largest safety margin during intraoperative testing. Final placement was confirmed with neuroimaging. Postoperatively, the optimal stimulation settings and antiparkinsonian medication were intermittently adjusted according to the patient's response. "Patients assigned to medical treatment received individualized optimal drug therapy according to the guidelines of the German Society of Neurology. The drugs were adjusted according to the patient's needs throughout the study."[2]

Follow-Up: All subjects underwent testing at baseline and at 6 months.

Endpoints: Primary outcome: changes from baseline to 6 months in the quality of life, as assessed by the Parkinson's Disease Questionnaire (PDQ-39) summary index, and in the severity of motor symptoms while the patient was not taking medication, as assessed by the Unified Parkinson's Disease Rating Scale, part III (UPDRS-III). Secondary outcome: changes in a Dyskinesia Scale and in the activities of daily living as assessed by the UDPRS, part II (UPDRS-II), and the Schwab and England Scale, with and without medication.

The PDQ-39 is used to assess well-being and functioning in Parkinson's patients and is completed by patients and their families.[3] It evaluates eight key dimensions:

- Mobility
- ADL
- Emotional well-being
- Stigma
- Social support
- Cognitions
- Communication
- Bodily discomfort

RESULTS

- Patients treated with neurostimulation had greater improvement in the score on the PDQ-39 summary index than did patients assigned to medical treatment (see Table 10.1).
- Patients treated with neurostimulation had greater improvement in the score on the UPDRS-III (to assess motor function) administered when the patients were not taking medication (see Table 10.1).
- ADLs while the patient was not taking medication, as assessed by the UPDRS-II, markedly improved in the neurostimulation group and slightly worsened in the medication group (see Table 10.1).
- Thirteen severe adverse events were reported in 13 patients (10 in the neurostimulation group and 3 in the medication group, $P = 0.04$). Three patients died in the deep-brain stimulation group: one from intracerebral hemorrhage during surgery, one from pneumonia 6 weeks after randomization, and one who committed suicide five months after randomization.

Table 10.1. Summary of Key Findings

Outcome Measures	Group				P Value
	Baseline Neurostimulation	Baseline Medication	Δ Baseline to 6 Mo Neurostimulation	Δ Baseline to 6 Mo Medication	
PDQ-39 Summary Index[a]	41.8 ± 13.9	39.6 ± 16.0	9.5 ± 15.3	−0.2 ± 11.2	0.02
UPDRS-III					
Without medication	48.0 ± 12.3	46.8 ± 12.1	19.6 ± 15.1	0.4 ± 9.5	<0.001
With medication	18.9 ± 9.3	17.3 ± 9.6	4.0 ± 10.1	−0.4 ± 7.7	0.01
UPDRS-II					
Without medication	22.5 ± 7.2	21.9 ± 6.4	8.8 ± 8.6	−0.8 ± 6.4	<0.001
With medication	9.0 ± 5.5	7.9 ± 5.8	1.5 ± 5.4	−1.1 ± 5.2	0.005
Dyskinesia Scale					
Without medication	0.5 ± 2.0	0.5 ± 1.7	0.2 ± 2.2	0.2 ± 1.7	0.78
With medication	6.7 ± 5.3	8.4 ± 5.9	3.4 ± 4.5	−0.4 ± 4.6	<0.001
Schwab and England Scale[b]					
Without medication	47 ± 19	48 ± 19	−23 ± 22	1 ± 16	<0.001
With medication	80 ± 19	82 ± 17	−4 ± 16	3 ± 16	0.02

[a] Scores for PDQ-39 can range from 0–100. Scores for UPDRS-III can range from 0–108. Scores for UPDRS-II can range from 0–52. Scores for the Dyskinesia Scale can range from 0–28. For all of these scales, lower scores indicate better function or quality of life.
[b] Scores for Schwab and England scale can range from 0–100. Higher scores indicate better function or quality of life.

Criticisms and Limitations: There was no sham-surgery or placebo control in this study. Multiple studies to date have demonstrated that neurostimulation of the subthalamic nucleus in Parkinson's disease is associated with a placebo effect. The implementation of a sham-surgery arm is controversial, however, because of its potential adverse effects. The best medical treatment group did not receive standardized therapy; rather, the choice of medication regimen was determined on an individual basis in accordance with national guidelines for the treatment of advanced Parkinson's disease, as published by the German Society of Neurology.

Other Relevant Studies and Information:

- This study primarily focused on quality of life measures, in contrast to previous studies, which used motor scales as the primary outcome measure.[4,5] These 2 studies demonstrated that subthalamic stimulation improved fluctuating motor symptoms; however, they were not prospective trials.
- The current guidelines on treating Parkinson's disease with motor fluctuations and dyskinesia were published by the American Academy of Neurology in 2006. They are compatible with this study and state, "DBS of the STN is possibly effective in improving motor function and reducing motor fluctuations, dyskinesia, and antiparkinsonian medication usage in [Parkinson's disease] patients."[6]

Summary and Implications: Subthalamic neurostimulation resulted in a signficant and clinically meaningful improvement in the quality of life of patients <75 years of age who had advanced Parkinson's disease with parkinsonian motor symptoms or dyskinesias. Patients who received neurostimulation had longer periods and better quality of mobility with less dyskinesia, compared to those patients who received best medical therapy alone.

CLINICAL CASE: MANAGEMENT OF ADVANCED PARKINSON'S DISEASE

Case History:
A 71-year-old woman with idiopathic Parkinson's disease diagnosed 10 years ago presents to clinic complaining of worsening mobility. She states that throughout the day she fluctuates between feeling stiff and slow just prior to her next dose of carbidopa-levodopa and experiencing uncontrollable dyskinesias. These symptoms interfere with her ability to perform many tasks, and her husband now helps with most of her ADL. Her parkinsonian symptoms have worsened despite escalation of medical therapy. She otherwise is healthy and takes one antihypertensive medication for high blood pressure. Both she and her husband report worsening quality of life and wonder if any other treatment options exist.

Suggested Answer:
This study demonstrated that deep-brain stimulation of the subthalamic nucleus in patients with advanced Parkinson's disease results in greater improvement in motor function and quality of life compared to best medical management.

The patient in this vignette has advanced Parkinson's disease, with severe motor fluctuations, despite optimal medical therapy. She has no evidence of dementia or major psychiatric illness and is otherwise healthy with no contraindications to surgery. Therefore, neurostimulation targeting the subthalamic nucleus should be recommended. Based on this study, neurostimulation is expected to improve her motor fluctuations, help her become more independent with her ADL, and improve her overall quality of life. Surgery is not without risks; however, for this patient the benefits of neurostimulation likely outweigh those risks, and DBS should be offered.

References

1. Deuschl G, Schade-Britinger C, Krack P, et al. A randomized trial of deep-brain stimulation for Parkinson's disease. *N Engl J Med.* 2006;355:896–908.
2. Oertel W, Deuschl G, Eggert K, et al. Parkinson-Syndrome. In: Diener HC, ed. Leitlinien für Diagnostik und Therapie in der Neurologie: Stuttgart: Thieme-Verlag, 2003:38–57.
3. Jenkinson C, Fitzpatrick R, Peto V, Greenhall R, Hyman N. The Parkinson's Disease Questionnaire (PDQ-39): development and validation of a Parkinson's disease summary index score. *Age Ageing.* 1997;26(5):353–357.

4. The Deep-Brain Stimulation for Parkinson's Disease Study Group. Deep-brain stimulation of the subthalamic nucleus or the pars interna of the globus pallidus in Parkinson's disease. *N Engl J Med.* 2001;345:956–63.
5. Krack P, Batir A, Van Blercom N, et al. Five-year follow-up of bilateral stimulation of the subthalamic nucleus in advanced Parkinson's disease. *N Engl J Med.* 2003;349:1925–1934.
6. Pahwa R, Factor SA, Lyons KE, et al. Practice parameter: Treatment of Parkinson disease with motor fluctuation and dyskinesia (an evidence-based review). *Neurology.* 2006;6:983–995.

SECTION VI

Multiple Sclerosis

11

Oral versus IV Steroids for Acute Relapses of Multiple Sclerosis

JOSHUA LOVINGER

> No difference in recovery . . . between the two treatment groups emerged at any stage of the trial.
> —BARNES ET AL.[1]

Research Question: Are oral steroids as effective as intravenous steroids in treatment of acute relapses of multiple sclerosis (MS)?[1]

Funding: Multiple Sclerosis Society of Great Britain and Northern Ireland.

Year Study Began: 1992

Year Study Published: 1997

Study Location: Guy's Hospital; the Royal London Hospital; Atkinson Morley's Hospital; Charing Cross Hospital; The National Hospital for Neurology and Neurosurgery, London; and the Queen Elizabeth Hospital, Birmingham.

Who Was Studied: Patients with "a relapse of MS within the previous 4 weeks severe enough to justify steroid treatment, age over 16 years, clinically definite MS (with MRI or evoked response evidence counting as a single lesion)."[1]

Who Was Excluded: Use of steroids or other immunosuppressive treatment during the previous month, pregnancy, inability to get informed consent from patient, or medical or psychiatric illness precluding steroid treatment.[1]

How Many Patients: 80

Study Overview: See Figure 11.1 for a summary of the trial design.

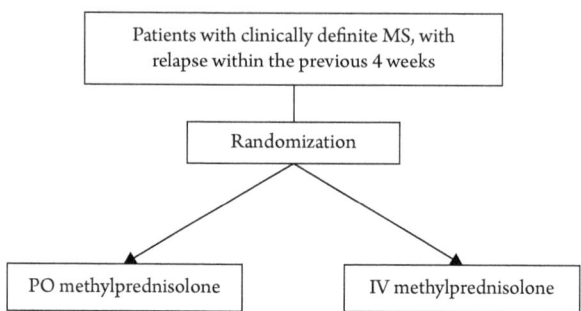

Figure 11.1 Summary of Trial Design.

Study Intervention: Patients randomized to the oral regimen received 48 mg methylprednisolone/day (equivalent to 60 mg prednisolone) in a single daily dose for 7 days, followed by 24 mg/day for 7 days, and finally 12 mg/day for 7 days. Patients randomized to the intravenous regimen received 1 g methylprednisolone a day given over 30 minutes on 3 consecutive days.

Follow-Up: Assessments were done at 1 week, 4 weeks, 12 weeks, and 24 weeks after randomization.

Endpoints: Primary outcome: Difference between the treatment groups in improvement in the Expanded Disability Status Scale of one or more grades 4 weeks after trial entry. The EDSS is scored 0–10 with 10 meaning most disability (0 = normal neurologic exam; 10 = death due to MS). The EDSS has an emphasis on mobility; cognitive effects of MS are notably underrepresented by EDSS. Secondary outcomes: (1) Difference of one or more grades in ambulation index 4 weeks after entry; (2) Difference of one or more grades in EDSS either 1 or 12 weeks after entry into the trial.

RESULTS

- After adjusting for baseline levels, the mean difference in EDSS at 4 weeks was 0.017 grades more in those taking oral steroids than in those on intravenous treatment. There were no significant differences between the two groups at any stage of the study (see Table 11.1).

Table 11.1. SUMMARY OF THE TRIAL'S KEY FINDINGS

Interval of Assessment	CHANGE IN MEDIAN EDSS (MEDIAN AND INTERQUARTILE RANGE)		P Value[a]
	IV Methylprednisolone (n = 38)	Oral Methylprednisolone (n = 42)	
Entry	6.0 (3.5–7.5)	5.0 (3.5–6.5)	—
Entry–1 week[b]	0 (0–0.5)	0.5 (0–1)	—
Entry–4 weeks[c]	0.5 (0–1.5)	0.5 (0–1.625)	0.80
Entry–12 weeks[b]	0.5 (0–1.5)	0.5 (0–1.5)	—
Entry–24 weeks	0.5 (0–1.5)	0.75 (0–1.5)	—

[a] P value was reported only for primary endpoint.
[b] Secondary endpoints.
[c] Primary endpoint.

Criticisms and Limitations: There was no standardization of what was considered a relapse. The criterion for inclusion was a relapse "severe enough to justify steroid treatment." This may differ between various patients and medical providers. No objective evidence of relapse, like imaging, was utilized.

The study excluded those patients who had used immunosuppressive treatment during the previous month. When the study was performed, there were no disease-modifying therapies (DMT) for MS on the market. In 1993, the first DMT, IFN beta-1b (Betaseron) was approved by the US FDA for relapsing-remitting MS. Today, most patients with clinically definite MS would likely be on immunomodulating therapy.

The population studied was atypical. For example, 75% (18/24) of the oral prednisone group was male, whereas other studies have typically reported a 3:1 female-to-male ratio for MS.[2] The course of MS in males and their response to therapy may differ from those of women.

Though the EDSS at time of study entry was similar between the two groups, a large proportion of patients who had high EDSS scores were included. Thirteen patients out of a study population of 80 (8/38 [21%] of the IV steroid group vs. 5/42 [19%] of the oral steroid group) had an EDSS ≥8, indicating severe disability. As Barkhof and Polman have noted,[3] the study population, by including a high number of patients with low or high EDSS scores, likely included a mix of relapsing-remitting and secondary progressive patients. Patients with progressive disease (potentially more numerous within the IV steroid group) likely would not respond to steroids.

Other Relevant Studies and Information:

- The Optic Neuritis Treatment Trial (ONTT)[4] was published while this study was conducted. Patients with optic neuritis received treatment for 14 days. They were assigned to (1) oral prednisone (1 mg/kg per day) for 14 days with a 4-day taper, (2) IV methylprednisolone (250 mg 4 times a day for 3 days, followed by oral prednisone for 11 days with a 4-day taper (a different IV protocol from Barnes et al.), or (3) oral placebo for 14 days. (For more on the ONTT, see Chapter 27.) Following publication of the ONTT, "with data suggesting that steroid therapy might influence subsequent relapse rate, at least in isolated optic neuritis, the protocol [for the study of Barnes et al.] was extended to record relapse and disability at 6 monthly intervals for 2 years after randomization."[5]
- A meta-analysis comparing oral and IV steroids for treatment of MS exacerbations also concluded that there is no significant difference between the route of administration of steroids and outcome.[6]

Summary and Implications: Oral steroids appear to be equally efficacious in treating MS exacerbations relative to IV steroids, are considerably cheaper, and do not require hospital admission. However, due to concerns about higher rates of recurrent optic neuritis with oral versus IV steroids based on other research (ONTT), some continue to prefer to treat MS flares with intravenous steroids.

CLINICAL CASE: ORAL VERSUS INTRAVENOUS METHYLPREDNISOLONE FOR ACUTE RELAPSES OF MULTIPLE SCLEROSIS

Case History:

A 35-year-old woman has been diagnosed with MS. She has had prior episodes of optic neuritis. She presents to your office within a week of onset of binocular horizontal diplopia with rightward gaze and a right facial droop. She has not had similar symptoms before. MRI of the brain with gadolinium demonstrates an enhancing lesion in the posterior pons near the facial colliculus. How should she be treated?

Suggested Answer:

The patient has a new, active MS lesion, consistent with an acute exacerbation. This trial and a later meta-analysis have shown a relative equivalence in outcome from treatment of such exacerbations with oral or intravenous steroids.

However, given the results of the ONTT, some would prefer to administer IV steroids based on an analogy between the new demyelinating lesion, regardless of the location, with optic neuritis (which has an increased recurrence rate when treated with oral vs. IV steroids).

References

1. Barnes D, Hughes RA, Morris RW, et al. Randomised trial of oral and intravenous methylprednisolone in acute relapses of multiple sclerosis. *Lancet.* 1997;349:902–906.
2. Orton SM, Herrera BM, Yee IM, et al. Sex ratio of multiple sclerosis in Canada: a longitudinal study. *Lancet Neurol.* 2006;5(11):932–936.
3. Barkhof F, Polman C. Oral or intravenous methylprednisolone for acute relapses of MS? *Lancet.* 1997;349(9056):893–894
4. Beck RW, Cleary PA, Anderson MM, et al. A randomized, controlled trial of corticosteroids in the treatment of acute optic neuritis. *NEJM.* 1992;326:581–588.
5. Sharrack B, Hughes RA, Morris RW, et al. The effect of oral and intravenous methylprednisolone treatment on subsequent relapse rate in multiple sclerosis. *J Neurol Sci.* 2000;173(1):73–77.
6. Burton JM, O'Connor PW, Hohol M, et al. Oral versus intravenous steroids for treatment of relapses in multiple sclerosis. *Cochrane Database Syst Rev.* 2012;12:CD006921.

12
Interferon Beta-1a for a First Demyelinating Event
The CHAMPS Trial
SARAH A. MULUKUTLA

> In our study, interferon beta-1a reduced the rate of development of clinically definite multiple sclerosis within three years by about half.
> —CHAMPS STUDY GROUP[1]

Research Question: Is interferon beta therapy beneficial when started soon after a patient's first clinical demyelinating event?[1]

Funding: Biogen Idec.

Year Study Began: 1996

Year Study Published: 2000

Study Location: 50 clinical centers in the United States and Canada.

Who Was Studied: Patients between 18–50 years old with (1) a first demyelinating event involving the optic nerve, spinal cord, brain stem, or cerebellum and (2) evidence of ≥2 clinically silent lesions on brain MRI.

Who Was Excluded: Patients with a prior neurologic or visual event that lasted >48 hours and patients who presented >14 days after the onset of clinical syndrome.

How Many Patients: 383

Study Overview: See Figure 12.1 for a summary of the trial design.

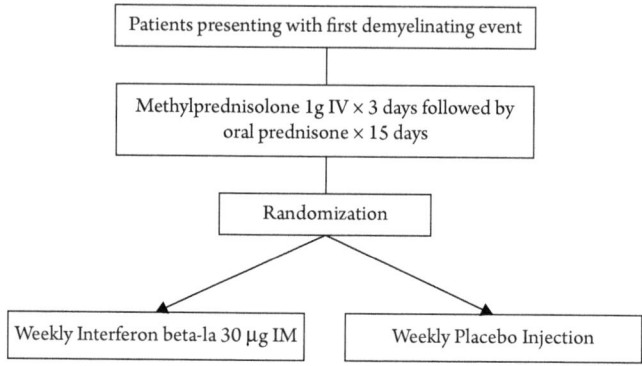

Figure 12.1 Summary of CHAMPS Design.

Study Intervention: Weekly intramuscular injection of interferon beta-1a 30 μg, or placebo, was administered for a planned duration of 3 years. To minimize symptoms of interferon-related influenza-like syndrome, all subjects were instructed to take acetaminophen 650 mg before each injection and every 6 hours × 24 hours during the first 6 months of treatment.

Follow-Up: 3 years. Physical examinations and laboratory assessments were made at months 1, 6, 12, 18, and 24. Brain MRI with and without gadolinium were performed at month 6, 12, and 18. At each visit, empty vials were counted to assess for medication compliance. If a patient reported a new visual or neurological symptom, clinical assessment was made within 7 days.

Endpoints: Primary outcome: clinically definite multiple sclerosis (CDMS). Conversion to CDMS was confirmed if patients had new neurologic symptoms lasting >48 hours with at least a 1.5-point increase in the score on the Expanded Disability Status Scale. If CDMS was confirmed, patients were withdrawn from the study and treatment was discontinued. Secondary outcomes: number of new or enlarging lesions on T2-weighted and number of gadolinium-enhancing lesions on T1-weighted MRI (see Table 12.1).

Table 12.1. SUMMARY OF MRI FINDINGS AT 18 MONTHS

Outcome	Treatment Group	Placebo Group	P Value
Mean change in volume of T2-weighted lesions (mm³)	28	313	<0.0001
Number of new or enlarging T2-weighted lesions	2.1 ± 3.2	5.0 ± 7.7	<0.0001
Number of gadolinium-enhancing T1-weighted lesions	0.4 ± 1.5	1.4 ± 3.6	<0.0001

RESULTS

- A predetermined interim analysis demonstrated significantly decreased disease activity in the treatment group, leading to early termination of the study in March 2000.
- Cumulative probability of developing CDMS during 3-year follow-up was 35% in treatment group versus 50% in placebo group ($P = 0.002$). Rate ratio for conversion was 0.56 in favor of the treatment group.
- Depression and flu-like syndrome were significantly more common in patients receiving the treatment medication versus placebo.
- Greater than 90% of subjects took the medication at least 80% of the time, suggesting good compliance for both groups.

Criticisms and Limitations: This trial does not provide data on the long-term benefits of early interferon beta-1a treatment, as patients were withdrawn from the study after developing CDMS.

Other Relevant Studies and Information:

- For patients with remitting-relapsing multiple sclerosis, prior studies had demonstrated efficacy of interferon beta in slowing the progression of physical disability, reducing the rate of clinical relapses, and reducing the development of brain lesions as shown on MRI.[2-4]
- After the CHAMPS study was published, subsequent studies have further demonstrated efficacy of early treatment with interferon beta-1a,[5] interferon beta-1b,[6] and glatiramer acetate[7] following first demyelinating event. Please see Chapter 13 for more information on the PreCISe study, in which early treatment with glatiramer acetate was investigated.
- The American Academy of Neurology and Multiple Sclerosis Council for Clinical Practice Guidelines name the CHAMPS study as class I evidence and supports early use of interferon beta-1a in any patient at high risk for developing CDMS.[8]

Summary and Implications: In patients at high risk for developing MS, early treatment with interferon beta-1a decreased the proportion of patients who converted to clinically definite disease by 44% in the first 3 years. Initiating treatment at first demyelinating event also reduced the accumulation rate of new MRI-detected white matter lesions during the 18 months of drug exposure. These results suggest that early initiation of disease-modifying treatment for first demyelinating events could have long-term benefits on disease progression, although long-term follow-up is necessary to confirm this hypothesis.

CLINICAL CASE: FIRST PRESENTATION OF A CLINICALLY ISOLATED DEMYELINATING EVENT

Case History:
A 32-year-old woman noted blurry vision in her left eye upon awakening one morning. Her vision continued to worsen for the next three days, prompting a visit to the local emergency room. She complained of retrobulbar pain when moving her eye, and felt that her vision worsened after a warm shower.

Ophthalmological examination revealed visual acuity 20/20 in the right eye, 20/100 in the left eye, together with an afferent pupillary defect on the left. She additionally reported decreased color saturation with the left eye. On fundoscopic exam, the patient's optic disc was swollen and pale. Her neurologic exam was otherwise normal. A diagnosis of optic neuritis was made.

MRI brain with and without contrast was obtained. Three lesions ranging from 3 mm–6 mm were seen in the bilateral cerebral hemispheres in typical ovoid form. No abnormal enhancement was seen.

Based on the CHAMPS study, what would the recommended therapy be for this patient?

Suggested Answer:
Methylprednisolone 1 g IV × 3 days is recommended as initial treatment for a clinically isolated event. After finishing the IV treatment, this patient would be a good candidate for early initiation of a disease-modifying agent to reduce the rate to development of CDMS, as she has evidence of prior demyelination on MRI. Weekly intramuscular interferon beta-1a was one of the first medications approved for patients with a first-time clinical demyelinating event, although several others have subsequently been approved.

References

1. Jacobs et al. Intramuscular interferon beta-1a therapy initiated during a first demyelinating event in multiple sclerosis. *N Engl J Med.* 2000;343(13):898–904.
2. Jacobs LD et al. Intramuscular interferon beta-1a for disease progression in relapsing multiple sclerosis. The Multiple Sclerosis Collaborative Research Group (MSCRG). *Ann Neurol.* 1996;39:285–294.
3. PRISMS (Prevention of Relapses and Disability by Interferon β-1a in relapsing/remitting multiple sclerosis). *Lancet.* 1998;352:1498–1504.
4. The IFNB Multiple Sclerosis Study Group. Interferon beta-1b is effective in relapsing-remitting multiple sclerosis. Clinical results of a multi-center, randomized, double-blind, placebo-controlled trial. *Neurology.* 1993;43:655–661.
5. Comi G et al. Effect of early interferon treatment on conversion to definite multiple sclerosis: a randomized study. *Lancet.* 2001;357:1576–1582.
6. Kappos et al. Treatment with interferon beta-1b delays conversion to clinically definite and McDonald MS in patients with clinically isolated syndromes. *Neurology.* 2006;67:1242–1249.
7. Comi G et al. Effect of glatiramer acetate on conversion to clinically definite multiple sclerosis in patients with clinically isolated syndrome (PreCISe study): a randomized, double-blind, placebo-controlled study. *Lancet.* 2009;374:1503–1511.
8. Therapeutics and Technology Assessment Subcommittee of the American Academy of Neurology and the MS Council for Clinical Practice Guidelines. Disease modifying therapies in multiple sclerosis. *Neurology.* 2002;58:169–178.

13

Glatiramer Acetate for Clinically Isolated Syndrome

The PreCISe Trial

SARAH A. MULUKUTLA

> [E]arly treatment with glatiramer acetate for patients with clinically isolated syndrome [a unifocal neurological event], who are at high risk for developing multiple sclerosis, significantly reduced the frequency of conversion to clinically definite [multiple sclerosis] and delayed the occurrence of a second attack.
>
> —Comi et al.[1]

Research Question: Previous data suggest that early treatment with interferon beta-1a or interferon beta-1b effectively delays onset to clinically definite multiple sclerosis (CDMS) in patients who experience a clinically isolated syndrome. Can early treatment with glatiramer acetate also reduce the risk of conversion to multiple sclerosis (MS) in these patients?[1]

Funding: Teva Pharmaceutical Industries, Israel.

Year Study Began: 2004

Year Study Published: 2009

Study Location: 16 countries worldwide, including 80 sites from the United States, Europe, Argentina, Australia, and New Zealand.

Who Was Studied: Patients aged between 18–45 years with a well-defined, single, unifocal neurological event (clinically isolated syndrome, CIS) and a brain MRI with at least two T2-weighted lesions measuring ≥6 mm, who presented within 90 days of attack onset.

Who Was Excluded: Patients with multifocal clinical presentation, those with diseases other than MS that might be responsible for the clinical or MRI presentation, use of experimental or investigational drugs, use of beta interferon or chronic corticosteroid treatment within 6 months of screening, a relapse between screening and enrollment visits, pregnancy or breastfeeding, and those with a known sensitivity to mannitol or gadolinium.

How Many Patients: 481

Study Overview: See Figure 13.1 for a summary of the trial's design.

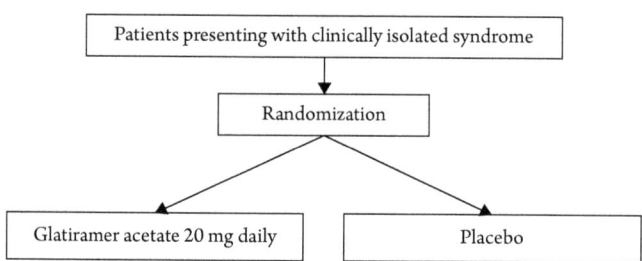

Figure 13.1 Summary of PreCISe Overview.

Study Intervention: After the initial clinical event, patients must not have taken corticosteroids (IV, IM, or PO) within 30 days prior to a baseline MRI for the study (per direct correspondence with manuscript authors). Treatment with daily, single-use, prefilled syringe containing 1 ml solution of 20 mg glatiramer acetate, 40 mg mannitol, and water for injection or a matching placebo was then initiated within 90 days of the CIS.

Follow-Up: Site visits at screening; randomization (baseline); months 1, 3, and every 3 months afterward; and at early termination. MR imaging with and without gadolinium at screening, baseline, and every 3 months thereafter until CDMS or completion of the 3-year placebo-controlled phase, and then every

6 months during a subsequent 2-year open-label phase. Mean exposure time during the prespecified interim analysis was 2.32 years.

Endpoints: Primary outcome: time to conversion to CDMS, consistent with the definition of MS relapse: an increase of ≥0.5 points on the Expanded Disability Status Scale (EDSS) or one grade in the score of 2 or more of the 7 Functional Systems (FS); or 2 grades in the score of one of the FS as compared to the previous evaluation. Secondary outcomes: number of new T2 lesions detected at last scan of the placebo-controlled phase (also called last observed value, or LOV); baseline-adjusted T2 lesions volume at LOV; brain atrophy, defined by percentage brain volume change from baseline scan to LOV; and proportion of patients who converted to CDMS during the placebo-controlled phase.

RESULTS

- At the time of interim analysis, 230/481 subjects (~48%) had completed the placebo-controlled phase of the trial (defined by conversion to CDMS or 3 years of exposure without a second clinical attack). Of 243 subjects assigned to glatiramer acetate, 98 had completed the study, 108 were still in the double-blind phase, and 37 terminated early. Of the 238 subjects assigned to placebo, 132 had completed the study, 85 were still in the double-blind phase, and 21 had terminated early.
- Among the 98 glatiramer acetate completers, 60 had converted to CDMS (61%). Of the 132 completers who received placebo, 102 had converted to CDMS (77%). This represented a 45% risk reduction in conversion to CDMS in the treatment group compared to the placebo group ($P = 0.0005$). Based on this finding, the study was discontinued and all subjects were transitioned to glatiramer acetate.
- The number needed to treat to prevent one patient from conversion to clinical definite multiple sclerosis is 5.49.
- The risk reduction was greatest in women, younger patients, and in patients with one or more gadolinium-enhancing lesions at entry into the study.
- With regard to adverse events, 56% of patients in the treatment group had injection site reactions compared with 24% in the placebo group. Other notable adverse events in the treatment group were vomiting (5.8%), lymphadenopathy (5.3%), and flu-like illness (4.1%).
- There was a larger number of patients in the treatment group compared to placebo who had early termination from the study (37/243 [15%] vs. 21/238 [9%], respectively).

- A statistically significant treatment effect of glatiramer acetate compared to placebo was demonstrated for two of the three MRI-related secondary endpoints (Table 13.1), including a reduction of 58% (rate ratio [95% CI]: 0.42 [0.29, 0.61], $P < 0.0001$) in the number of new T2 lesions at LOV of the placebo-controlled phase.

Table 13.1. SUMMARY OF ADDITIONAL PreCISe's FINDINGS

Outcome	Treatment Group	Placebo Group	P value
Days to relapse in fastest quartile of patients converting to CDMS	722	336	0.005
Proportion of subjects who had a second attack within 3 years of treatment (%)	24.7	42.9	<0.0001
Number of new T2 lesions at LOV	0.7	1.8	<0.0001
Cumulative number of new T2 lesions at LOV	4.2	9.8	<0.0001

Criticisms and Limitations: The study's secondary outcomes, which involve counting lesions on MRI at LOV, potentially could be biased against active treatment because patients in the treatment group had a longer time period leading up to LOV. To address this limitation, all scans available up to 12 months and 24 months were factored into the analysis for subjects who did not convert to CDMS. Of note, this was a placebo-controlled protocol that passed institutional review boards despite the availability of interferons as a treatment option for CIS.

Other Relevant Studies and Information:

- Results of the subsequent open-label phase of the PreCISe trial were published in 2013 and demonstrated benefit of early versus delayed treatment with glatiramer acetate with continued follow-up.[2]
- The range of efficacy of glatiramer acetate was similar to the efficacy of early treatment with interferon beta-1a[3] and interferon beta-1b.[4,5]
- Guidelines published by the American Academy of Neurology and the Multiple Sclerosis Council for Clinical Practice advocate the use of early treatment of disease-modifying agents for patients at high risk for developing CDMS.[6] The most recent guidelines published in 2002 do not include glatiramer acetate as they were published prior to the PreCISe trial. Since then, glatiramer acetate has received approval for use in CIS.

Summary and Implications: This study demonstrated that early treatment with glatiramer acetate in patients with CIS significantly delays time to onset of CDMS. The drug was tolerated by most participants, and efficacy was similar to that of the interferons. Patients who are at risk for developing multiple sclerosis should be placed on disease-modifying treatment as early as possible. Glatiramer acetate for CIS is a favorable option because of its mild side effect profile.

CLINICAL CASE: FIRST PRESENTATION OF A CLINICALLY ISOLATED EVENT

Case History:
A 24-year-old woman presents to her physician with 1 week of difficulty walking due to left leg weakness. She complains of tripping, leg buckling, and dragging her foot. She denies sensory changes, weakness in other extremity, bowel or bladder incontinence, or change in vision. She has never had neurologic deficits like this before. There is no family history of multiple sclerosis.

An MRI brain with and without contrast is ordered, which reveals 9 T2-weighted hyperintense lesions of varying size scattered throughout the cerebrum. They occur in both cerebral hemispheres, and 3 are perpendicular to the corpus callosum on sagittal views. One lesion in the right frontal lobe enhances with gadolinium.

Based on the PreCISe study, is glatiramer acetate indicated for this 24-year-old patient?

Suggested Answer:
After corticosteroid therapy is complete, initiation of a disease-modifying agent is indicated for this young patient with high risk for conversion to CDMS. Glatiramer acetate 20 mg daily subcutaneous injection is one option that has been shown to effectively delay onset to a second clinical attack. Other options include interferon beta-1a and interferon beta-1b.

References

1. Comi G, Martinelli V, Rodegher M, et al. Effect of glatiramer acetate on conversion to clinically definite multiple sclerosis in patients with clinically isolated syndrome (PreCISe study): a randomized, double-blind, placebo-controlled trial. *Lancet.* 2009;374:1503–1511.

2. Comi G, Martinelli V, Rodegher M, et al. Effects of early treatment with glatiramer acetate in patients with clinically isolated syndrome. *Mult Scler.* 2013; 19(8):1074–1083.
3. Jacobs LD, Beck RW, Simon JH, et al. Intramuscular interferon beta-1a therapy initiated during a first demyelinating event in multiple sclerosis. *N Engl J Med.* 2000;323(12):898–904.
4. Comi G, Filippi M, Barkhof F, et al. Effect of early interferon treatment on conversion to definite multiple sclerosis: a randomised study. *Lancet.* 2001;357(9268): 1576–1582.
5. Kappos L, Polman CH, Freedman MS, et al. Treatment with interferon beta-1b delays conversion to clinically definite and McDonald MS in patients with clinically isolated syndromes. *Neurology.* 2006;67(7):1242–1249.
6. Therapeutics and Technology Assessment Subcommittee of the American Academy of Neurology and the MS Council for Clinical Practice Guidelines. Disease modifying therapies in multiple sclerosis. *Neurology.* 2002;58:169–178.

Natalizumab for Relapsing Multiple Sclerosis

The SENTINEL Trial

ROBERT J. CLAYCOMB

> Natalizumab added to interferon beta-1a was significantly more effective than interferon beta-1a alone in patients with relapsing multiple sclerosis.... [however,] two cases of progressive multifocal leukoencephalopathy, one of which was fatal, were diagnosed in the ... [dual-therapy] patients.
>
> —RUDICK ET AL.[1]

Research Question: Despite treatment with disease-modifying agents such as interferon beta and glatiramer acetate, most patients with multiple sclerosis (MS) still have relapses.[2,3] Previous studies have suggested that natalizumab (an α_4 integrin antagonist) may be both safe and effective for decreasing the incidence of MS relapses.[4] Is natalizumab in combination with interferon therapy associated with fewer relapses in patients with relapsing-remitting MS (RRMS) when compared to interferon therapy alone?[1]

Funding: Supported by Biogen Idec and Elan Pharmaceuticals.

Year Study Began: 2002

Year Study Published: 2006

Study Location: 124 sites within the United States and Europe

Who Was Studied: Patients aged 18–55 years with an MRI-confirmed diagnosis of RRMS. Additionally, patients needed to receive interferon beta-1a therapy for the 12 months preceding trial entry, during which time the patient needed to have had at least one exacerbation on therapy.

Who Was Excluded: Other forms of MS were excluded, including primary progressive, secondary progressive, and progressive relapsing MS. Also, patients were excluded if they experienced an exacerbation within 50 days of randomization or had received another type of disease-modifying therapy other than interferon beta-1a.

How Many Patients: 1,196

Study Overview: See Figure 14.1 for a summary of the trial design.

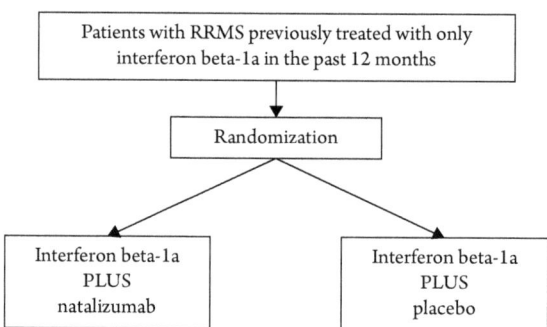

Figure 14.1 Summary of SENTINEL Design.

Study Intervention: Patients were randomized to receive either 300 mg of natalizumab or placebo intravenously every 4 weeks in addition to 30 μg of interferon beta-1a intramuscularly every week for up to 116 weeks.

Follow-Up: 120 weeks. Patients were seen by an examining neurologist every 12 weeks (who performed a neurological exam and administered the Expanded Disability Status Scale [EDSS] but did not participate in other aspects of care) and a treating neurologist who managed all aspects of care including relapses and adverse events.

Endpoints: Primary efficacy endpoints: the rate of new clinical relapses at 1 year and the cumulative probability of sustained disability progression at 2 years. New relapses were defined as new or recurrent neurological symptoms that (1) were not associated with an infection, (2) lasted greater than 24 hours, and (3) were associated with new and objective neurological findings. Sustained disability progression was defined as either (1) an increase by ≥1.0 point in the EDSS score if the baseline score was ≥1.0 or (2) an increase by ≥1.5 points in the EDSS if the baseline score was 0.0 and the increased score had to be sustained for greater than 12 weeks.

Secondary endpoints: the appearance of new or enlargement of old T2-hyperintense lesions on brain MRI and the appearance of gadolinium-enhancing lesions on MRI brain.

RESULTS

- "The hazard ratio for sustained progression in the combination-therapy group as compared with the group given interferon beta-1a alone was 0.76 (95% confidence interval, 0.6 to 0.96)"[1] (Table 14.1)
- During the course of the study, persistent anti-natalizumab antibodies (antibodies that were detected more than twice, over 41 days apart) were found in 38 (6%) of natalizumab-treated patients. (Table 14.2)

Table 14.1. SUMMARY OF KEY FINDINGS

Endpoint	Natalizumab Group	Placebo Group	P Value
Annualized relapse rate at 1 year[a]	0.38	0.81	<0.001
Cumulative 2-year probability of sustained disease progression[b]	23%	29%	0.02
Number of new or enlarging T2 hyperintense lesions after 2 years[b]	0.9 ± 2.1	5.4 ± 8.7	<0.001
Number of gadolinium-enhancing lesions after 2 years[c]	0.1 ± 0.4	0.9 ± 3.2	<0.001

[a] The annualized relapse rate per year was calculated as the total number of relapses divided by the number of subject-years.
[b] Sustained disability progression was defined as either (1) an increase by ≥1.0 point in the EDSS score if the baseline score was ≥1.0 or (2) an increase by ≥1.5 points in the EDSS if the baseline score was 0.0 and the increased score had to be sustained for greater than 12 weeks.
[c] Values are mean ± standard deviation.

Table 14.2. ADVERSE EVENTS

Adverse Event	Natalizumab Group	Placebo Group	P Value
Anxiety	12%	8%	≤0.01
Pharyngitis	7%	4%	≤0.05
Sinus congestion	6%	3%	≤0.01
Peripheral edema	5%	1%	≤0.001
Progressive multifocal leukoencephalopathy (PML)*	<1%	0%	>0.05

* There were 2 confirmed cases of PML in the natalizumab group. One occurred during the 2-year treatment period, and one after the conclusion of the 2-year study while the patient was in the extension study. A third case of PML was found retrospectively from a natalizumab trial in Crohn disease that had originally been misdiagnosed as astrocytoma.

Criticisms and Limitations: The study was stopped a few weeks prematurely in February 2005 and the use of natalizumab was temporarily suspended after cases of progressive multifocal leukoencephalopathy (PML) were linked to the use of natalizumab.

More than 80% of patients, regardless of treatment group, were fully ambulatory without the need for assistive devices and only had minimal to moderate functional disability. Therefore, this study excluded more advanced MS cases, and the efficacy of natalizumab in these cases was not addressed.

Only patients with relapsing-remitting MS were included, and the efficacy of natalizumab in other subtypes of MS was not addressed.

Other Relevant Studies and Information:

- The AFFIRM trial demonstrated that natalizumab monotherapy was also associated with delayed progression of RRMS and fewer T2 hyperintense lesions on MRI brain.[5] No cases of PML linked to natalizumab monotherapy were found.
- Currently natalizumab monotherapy (as opposed to combined therapy as in the SENTINEL study) is the only FDA-approved use of natalizumab for RRMS.
- The most current American Academy of Neurology Guidelines reserve the use of natalizumab monotherapy for the most refractory cases of RRMS.[6]

- The actual risk of natalizumab-associated PML was estimated to be about 1/1,000 cases in a study by Yousry et al.[7] That study examined over 3,300 patients who had received natalizumab as a part of a clinical trial (with or without other disease-modifying treatments) and found no additional confirmed cases of PML and only one indeterminate case.[7]

Summary and Implications: Natalizumab in addition to interferon beta-1a therapy is associated with a slower progression of RRMS. However, the use of natalizumab in combination with interferon beta-1a was associated with PML.[1] Regardless of its low PML risk, use of natalizumab monotherapy is limited only to patients with treatment-refractory RRMS.

CLINICAL CASE: NATALIZUMAB AND RELAPSING-REMITTING MULTIPLE SCLEROSIS

Case History:

A 29-year-old woman with a 5-year history of RRMS presents for routine follow-up. She was initially diagnosed after developing persistent diplopia. She has relapses about twice a year requiring in-patient hospitalization for intravenous corticosteroids. About 3 years ago, she was started on interferon beta-1a and has tolerated this well. Besides her mild diplopia she has no other disabilities and lives completely independently with her husband and two children. She also has a history of mild anxiety and depression that has been well controlled with daily paroxetine.

Her examination is notable for a right intranuclear ophthalmoplegia and mild increased tone in her left leg. Her EDSS score is 0.0 (no deficits). A serum test for anti-JC virus antibodies is negative. Her brain MRI reveals no gadolinium-enhancing lesions, but there are 22 distinct T2-hyperintense lesions involving the right juxtacortical frontal lobe, the bilateral periventricular areas, and the midbrain.

Should this patient be switched to natalizumab monotherapy?

Suggested Answer:

No. The patient's clinical course has not appreciably deteriorated in the past few years and is relatively stable. Despite a low risk of PML given her lack of JC virus antibodies (suggesting there is no latent JC viral infection) treatment with natalizumab still represents an unnecessary risk. She should continue with her interferon beta-1a therapy.

References

1. Rudick RA, Stuart WH, Calabresi PA, et al. Natalizumab plus interferon beta-1a for relapsing multiple sclerosis. *N Engl J Med.* 2006;354(9):911–923.
2. The IFNB Multiple Sclerosis Study Group. Interferon beta-1b is effective in relapsing-remitting multiple sclerosis. I. Clinical results of a multicenter, randomized, double-blind, placebo-controlled trial. *Neurology.* 1993;43(4):655–661.
3. PRISMS Study Group. Randomised double-blind placebo-controlled study of interferon beta-1a in relapsing/remitting multiple sclerosis. *Lancet.* 1998;352(9139):1498–1504.
4. Miller DH, Khan OA, Sheremata WA, et al. A controlled trial of natalizumab for relapsing multiple sclerosis. *N Engl J Med.* 2003;348(1):15–23.
5. Polman CH, O'Connor PW, Havrdova E, et al. A randomized, placebo-controlled trial of natalizumab for relapsing multiple sclerosis. *N Engl J Med.* 2006;354(9):899–910.
6. Goodin DS, Cohen BA, O'Connor P, Kappos L, Stevens JC; Therapeutics and Technology Assessment Subcommittee of the American Academy of Neurology. Assessment: the use of natalizumab (Tysabri) for the treatment of multiple sclerosis (an evidence-based review): report of the Therapeutics and Technology Assessment Subcommittee of the American Academy of Neurology. *Neurology.* 2008;71(10):766–773.
7. Yousry TA, Major EO, Ryschkewitsch C, et al. Evaluation of patients treated with natalizumab for progressive multifocal leukoencephalopathy. *N Engl J Med.* 2006;354(9):924–933.

15

Fingolimod for Relapsing Multiple Sclerosis

The TRANSFORMS Trial

MARY A. BAILEY

> This trial showed the superior efficacy of oral fingolimod . . . , as compared with intramuscular interferon beta-1a.
>
> —COHEN ET AL.[1]

Research Question: Does oral fingolimod, a sphingosine-1-phosphate receptor modulator that sequesters lymphocytes in lymph nodes, or intramuscular interferon have superior efficacy in treating relapsing multiple sclerosis?[1]

Funding: Novartis Pharmaceuticals.

Year Study Began: 2006

Year Study Published: 2010

Study Location: 172 clinical centers worldwide, including 37 in the United States.

Who Was Studied: Patients aged 18–55 years with clinically definite relapsing-remitting multiple sclerosis (RRMS) who had experienced one relapse within the past year or two relapses within the past 2 years and had an Expanded Disability Status Scale (EDSS) score of between 0–5.5.[2] Previous therapy with either interferon beta or glatiramer acetate was permitted.

Who Was Excluded: Patients who experienced a relapse or were treated with corticosteroids within 30 days of randomization. Other exclusion criteria included active infection, macular edema, immunosuppression, and significant other systemic disease or illness.

How Many Patients: 1,292

Study Overview: See Figure 15.1 for a summary of the study design.

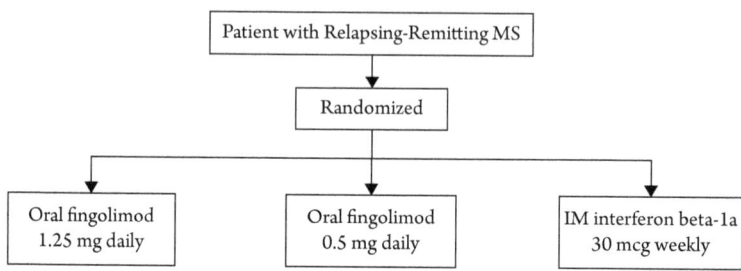

Figure 15.1 Summary of Study Design.

Study Intervention: Patients with clinically definite RRMS relapse were randomized to either receive oral fingolimod at 1.25 mg daily, oral fingolimod at 0.5 mg daily, or intramuscular interferon beta-1a 30 mcg weekly with a double-blind, double-dummy design.

Follow-Up: 12 months.

Endpoints: Primary outcome: number of confirmed relapses during a 12-month period. Secondary outcomes: time to disability progression; number of new or enlarged T2 weighted hyperintense lesions on MRI scans. Safety assessments were performed at baseline, months 1, 2, 3, 6, 9, and 12. EDSS was assessed every 3 months, while Multiple Sclerosis Functional Composite (MSFC) scores were performed every 6 months. The MSFC battery of tests includes a timed 25-foot walk, a 9-hole peg test, and a serial-addition task. MRI scans were done at screening and at month 12.

RESULTS

- In both groups who received fingolimod, the annualized relapse rates and lesion activity on MRI were reduced compared to the intramuscular interferon beta-1a group (see Table 15.1).

- The lower dose of fingolimod was at least as effective as the higher dose within the 12-month study period.
- There were no significant differences in progression of disability among the three groups.
- In the high-dose fingolimod group (1.25 mg daily), there were two fatal infections, one each caused by herpes simplex encephalitis and disseminated varicella zoster.
- Some of the other important adverse events seen in both fingolimod groups included bradycardia, atrioventricular block, macular edema, transaminitis, and nonfatal herpes virus infections.
- The most common adverse events in the interferon beta-1a group included influenza-like symptoms, pyrexia, myalgias, and depression.

Table 15.1. TRANSFORMS: CLINICAL AND MRI RESULTS AT 12 MONTHS

	FINGOLIMOD		Interferon Beta-1a (n = 431)	P VALUE	
	1.25 mg (n = 420)	0.5 mg (n = 429)		Fingolimod 1.25 mg vs. Interferon Beta-1a	Fingolimod 0.5 mg vs. Interferon Beta-1a
Annualized relapse rate (primary end point)—no. (95% CI)	0.20 (0.16–0.26)	0.16 (0.12–0.21)	0.33 (0.26–0.42)	<0.001	<0.001
MRI outcome	1.5 ± 2.7	1.7 ± 3.9	2.6 ± 5.8	<0.001	0.004
Disability Patients with no confirmed disability progression—% (95% CI)	93.3 (90.9–95.8)	94.1 (91.8–96.3)	92.1 (89.4–94.7)	0.5	0.25

Criticisms and Limitations: The follow-up for this study was only 12 months, which makes conclusions regarding disability outcomes difficult. Also, because this study was only 12 months in duration, there may be some late-appearing adverse events that may not have been detected. For example, in the fingolimod groups there were 10 localized skin cancers identified, 8 within 4 to 12 months after enrollment. There were also 4 cases of breast cancer diagnosed in the fingolimod groups, 3 being diagnosed within 4 months of drug initiation and 1 diagnosed 11 months after enrollment. These malignancies, and their possible association with treatment, need to be further investigated over a longer duration.

Other Relevant Studies and Information:

- Multiple other studies have demonstrated similar results to TRANSFORMS with regard to reduction in relapse rate and MRI outcomes, though these studies compare fingolimod to placebo.
- They have also demonstrated similar adverse events for fingolimod. One study looked at subgroups of patients treated with fingolimod (each subgroup characterized by similar degrees of disease activity in treatment–naïve or previously treated patients), and found it to be effective among a range of disease severity and baseline MRI characteristics (T2 lesion volume and number of gadolinium-enhancing lesions at baseline).[3–7]

Summary and Implications: In patients with RRMS, oral fingolimod is superior to intramuscular interferon beta-1a with regard to relapse rates and MRI outcomes. Therefore, fingolimod can be a good treatment option for patients who have had disease breakthrough activity, who do not tolerate interferon beta-1a or other disease modifying therapies, or as initial therapy.

CLINICAL CASE: FINGOLIMOD FOR RELAPSING MULTIPLE SCLEROSIS

Case History:
A 43-year-old woman with RRMS has been treated with intramuscular interferon beta-1a for the past 5 years. She tolerates the drug well and has had clinically and radiologically stable disease activity. However, she states she is tired of having to give herself injections. She comes to the office complaining of new weakness in the right leg. She has never had this symptom before and is very concerned because it is affecting her gait. She undergoes an MRI that demonstrates a new, enhancing thoracic spinal cord lesion. Given this new disease activity, how would you change her long-term MS treatment plan?

Suggested Answer:
Because she is having an acute relapse with a new lesion in her spinal cord, this is considered breakthrough disease activity, placing her at risk for future disability. There are many options for how to proceed with her long-term treatment, but she does express a dislike of self-injections. Therefore, given the data of the superior efficacy of oral fingolimod to intramuscular interferon beta-1a with regard to relapse rates and MRI findings, she could switch to treatment with oral fingolimod.

References

1. Cohen JA, Barkhof F, Comi G, et al. Oral fingolimod or intramuscular interferon for relapsing multiple sclerosis. *N Engl J Med.* 2010;362:402–415.
2. Kurtzke JF. Rating neurologic impairment in multiple sclerosis: an expanded disability status scale (EDSS). *Neurology.* 1983;33(11):1444–1452.
3. O'Connor P, Comi G, Montalban X, et al. Oral fingolimod (FTY720) in multiple sclerosis: two-year results of a phase II extension study. *Neurology.* 2009; 72(1):73–79.
4. Izquierdo G, O'Connor P, Montalban X, et al. Five-year results from a phase 2 study of oral fingolimod in relapsing multiple sclerosis. *Mult Scler.* 2013 Nov 30. [Epub ahead of print]
5. Devonshire V, Havrdova E, Radue EW, et al. Relapse and disability outcomes in patients with multiple sclerosis treated with fingolimod: subgroup analyses of the double-blind, randomized, placebo-controlled FREEDOMS study. *Lancet Neurol.* 2012;11(5):420–428
6. Kappos L, Antel J, Comi G, et al. Oral fingolimod (FTY720) for relapsing multiple sclerosis. *N Engl J Med.* 2006;355(11):1124–1140.
7. Kappos L, Radue EW, O'Connor P, et al. A placebo-controlled trial of oral fingolimod in relapsing multiple sclerosis. *N Engl J Med.* 2010;362:387–401.

16

Oral BG-12 for Relapsing-Remitting Multiple Sclerosis, Part I

The DEFINE Trial

MARY A. BAILEY

> ... BG-12, as compared with placebo, significantly reduced the proportion of patients who had a relapse by 2 years, the annualized rate of relapse, and the cumulative progression of disability.
>
> —Gold et al.[1]

Research Question: Is oral BG-12, dimethyl fumarate, a safe and efficacious for treatment of relapsing-remitting multiple sclerosis (RRMS) compared to placebo?[1]

Funding: Biogen Idec.

Year Study Began: 2007

Year Study Published: 2012

Study Location: 198 sites in 28 countries.

Who Was Studied: Adults aged 18–55 years with clinically definite RRMS who had an Expanded Disability Status Scale (EDSS) score between 0 and 5.0 (range 1–10, with higher score = more disability). All enrolled patients had a clinical relapse within the 12 months prior to enrollment, or at least one gadolinium-enhancing lesion on MRI within 6 weeks of enrollment.

Who Was Excluded: Patients with progressive forms of multiple sclerosis (MS), other significant medial comorbidities, prespecified laboratory abnormalities, or exposure to contraindicated medications.

How Many Patients: 1,237 randomized, 1,234 included in the intention-to-treat population.

Study Overview: See Figure 16.1 for a summary of the study design.

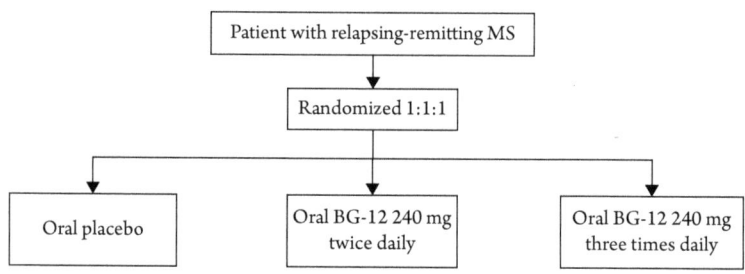

Figure 16.1 Summary of Study Design for DEFINE.

Study Intervention: Patients with RRMS were randomized in a double-blind fashion to an oral placebo, oral BG-12 240 mg twice daily, or oral BG-12 240 mg three times daily. Because BG-12 can cause flushing, all patients taking oral study medication were instructed to not take their medication within 4 hours of a study visit so that blinding was preserved.

Follow-Up: Mean follow-up of 83.9 weeks for all 3 groups.

Endpoints: The primary outcome was the proportion of patients who experienced a relapse by 2 years. Symptoms for relapses had to last at least 24 hours. Secondary outcomes included new lesions on MRI, annualized relapse rates, and time to progression of disability (i.e., 1-point increase in the EDSS with a baseline score ≥1.0, or a 1.5-point increase with a baseline score of 0).

RESULTS

- Both active treatment groups had a lower proportion of patients with relapses, a lower proportion of patients with progression of disability, a lower annualized relapse rate, and fewer numbers of new or enlarging lesions on MRI compared to the placebo group (see Table 16.1).

Table 16.1. DEFINE: BG-12 AS COMPARED TO PLACEBO

	Twice-daily BG-12	Thrice-daily BG-12
Frequency of relapses: annualized relapse rate ratio at 2 years vs. placebo	53% ($P < 0.001$)	48% ($P < 0.001$)
Disability progression: hazard ratio vs. placebo	0.62	0.66
Percent reduction of number of new or enlarged hyperintense lesions on T2-weighted images at 2 years vs. placebo	85% ($P < 0.001$)	74% ($P < 0.001$)

Criticisms and Limitations: DEFINE was a placebo-controlled trial in an era of MS care in which effective disease-modifying therapies exist. This potentially could be viewed as unethical since patients in the placebo arm of the studies were at risk of uncontrolled disease activity. However, placebo-controlled trials are still the gold standard trial design when assessing efficacy and safety of a treatment and are approved in the context of the following: (1) when patients refuse established, effective therapies; (2) have not responded to them; or (3) are unable to obtain them (e.g., for economic reasons).[2]

Other Relevant Studies and Information:

- Subgroup analyses have been done on the effectiveness and safety of oral BG-12 and have similar findings to the studies just discussed.[3-5]

Summary and Implications: In patients with RRMS, oral BG-12 has been shown to be an effective disease-modifying therapy versus placebo. This finding gives physicians and patients more options for MS treatments than the established injectable therapies.

CLINICAL CASE: ORAL BG-12 FOR RELAPSING MULTIPLE SCLEROSIS

Please refer to the case at the end of Chapter 17.

References

1. Gold R, Kappos L, Arnold DL, et al. Placebo-controlled phase 3 study of oral BG-12 for relapsing multiple sclerosis. *N Engl J Med*. 2012;367:1098–1107
2. Polman CH, Reingold SC, Barkhof F, et al. Ethics of placebo-controlled trials in multiple sclerosis: a reassessment. *Neurol*. 2008;70(13 Pt 2):1134–1140.
3. Kappos L, Gold R, Miller DH, et al. Efficacy and safety of oral fumarate in patients with relapsing-remitting multiple sclerosis: a multicentre, randomized, double-blind, placebo-controlled phase IIb study. *Lancet*. 2008;372(9648):1463–1472.
4. Havrdova E, Hutchinson M, Kurukulasuriya NC, et al. Oral BG-12 (dimethyl fumarate) for relapsing-remitting multiple sclerosis: a review of DEFINE and CONFIRM. Evaluation of: Gold R, Kappos L, Arnold D, et al. Placebo-controlled phase 3 study of oral BG-12 for relapsing multiple sclerosis. N Engl J Med 2012;367:1098-107; and Fox RJ, Miller DH, Phillips JT, et al. Placebo-controlled phase 3 study of oral BG-12 or glatiramer in multiple sclerosis. N Engl J Med 2012;367:1087-97. *Expert Opin Pharmacother*. 2013;14(15):2145–2156.
5. Bar-Or A, Gold R, Kappos L, et al. Clinical efficacy of BG-12 (dimethyl fumarate) in patients with relapsing-remitting multiple sclerosis: subgroup analyses of the DEFINE study. *J Neurol*. 2013;260(9):2297–2305.

Oral BG-12 for Relapsing-Remitting Multiple Sclerosis, Part II

The CONFIRM Trial

MARY A. BAILEY

> ... BG-12 (at both doses) and glatiramer acetate significantly reduced relapse rates and improved neuroradiologic outcomes relative to placebo.
> —Fox et al.[1]

Research Question: Is oral BG-12, dimethyl fumarate, safe and efficacious for treatment of relapsing-remitting multiple sclerosis (RRMS) compared to placebo and injectable glatiramer acetate?[1]

Funding: Biogen Idec.

Year Study Began: 2007

Year Study Published: 2012

Study Location: 200 sites in 28 countries.

Who Was Studied: Adults aged 18–55 years with clinically definite RRMS who had an Expanded Disability Status Scale (EDSS) between 0 and 5.0

(range 1–10, with higher score = more disability). All enrolled patients had a clinical relapse within the 12 months prior to enrollment, or at least one gadolinium-enhancing lesion on MRI between within 6 weeks of enrollment.

Who Was Excluded: Patients with progressive forms of multiple sclerosis (MS), other significant medial comorbidities, prespecified laboratory abnormalities, or prior exposure to glatiramer acetate or other contraindicated medications.

How Many Patients: 1,430 randomized, 1,417 evaluated in the intention-to-treat population.

Study Overview: See Figure 17.1 for a summary of the study design.

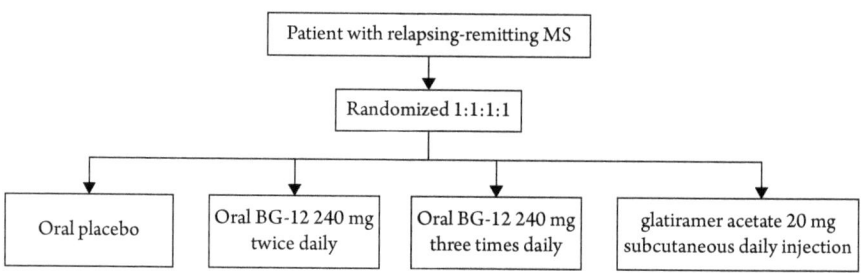

Figure 17.1 Summary of Study Design for CONFIRM.

Study Intervention: Patients with RRMS were randomized in a double-blind fashion to an oral placebo, oral BG-12 240 mg twice daily, or oral BG-12 240 mg three times daily. A fourth group of patients who was randomly assigned to treatment with glatiramer acetate 20 mg daily subcutaneous injections. These patients were *not* blinded. Because BG-12 can cause flushing, all patients taking oral study medication were instructed to not take their medication within 4 hours of a study visit so that blinding was preserved.

Follow-Up: Mean follow-up was 86.1, 84.4, 84.1, and 88.5 weeks in the placebo, twice daily BG-12, thrice daily BG-12, and glatiramer acetate groups, respectively.

Endpoints: The primary outcome was the annualized relapse rates. Secondary outcomes were new lesions on MRI, the proportion of patients with a relapse at 2 years, and the time to progression of disability at 2 years.

RESULTS

- At 2 years, the rate of relapse, the proportion of patients with a relapse, and MRI disease activity were each lower in all three active treatment arms of the study compared to placebo. None of the treatment groups demonstrated a significant effect on disability progression, unlike the effect seen for both BG-12 groups in DEFINE.[2] The most common adverse events in the BG-12 groups include flushing and gastrointestinal symptoms (see Table 17.1).
- In a post-hoc analysis of CONFIRM, three different measures revealed a greater treatment effect of BG-12 when directly compared to glatiramer acetate: annualized relapse rate, the number of new hypointense lesions on T1-weighted imaging (with thrice-daily BG-12), and the number of new or enlarging hyperintense lesions on T2-weighted imaging (with both BG-12 doses).

Table 17.1. CONFIRM: BG-12 AS COMPARED TO GLATIRAMER ACETATE

	Twice-daily BG-12	Thrice-daily BG-12	Glatiramer Acetate
Frequency of relapses: Percent reduction of annualized relapse rate at 2 years vs. placebo	44% ($P < 0.001$)	51% ($P < 0.001$)	29% ($P = 0.01$)
Relative reduction of disability progression vs. placebo	21% ($P = 0.25$)	24% ($P = 0.2$)	7% ($P = 0.7$)
Percent reduction of mean number of new or enlarged hyperintense lesions on T2-weighted images at 2 years vs. placebo	71% ($P < 0.001$)	73% ($P < 0.001$)	54% ($P < 0.001$)

Criticisms and Limitations:

- CONFIRM was a placebo-controlled trial in an era of MS care in which effective disease-modifying therapies exist. This potentially could be viewed as unethical since patients in the placebo arm of the studies were at risk of uncontrolled disease activity. However, placebo-controlled trials are still the gold standard trial design when assessing efficacy and safety of a treatment and are approved in the context of the following: (1) when patients refuse established, effective therapies; (2) have not responded to them; or (3) are unable to obtain them (e.g., economical reasons).[3] A limitation of CONFIRM is the post-hoc analysis comparing BG-12 to glatiramer acetate. This trial was designed with glatiramer as a reference group and not to directly compare these two treatments; thus it is premature to assume validity of the results of an underpowered post-hoc analysis. Of note, the lack of a significant effect of BG-12 on disability progression in CONFIRM may be due to the fact that the percentage of patients in the placebo group who had disability progression (17%) was significantly lower than in the placebo group for DEFINE (27%).

Other Relevant Studies and Information:

- Subgroup analyses have been done on the effectiveness and safety of oral BG-12, and have similar findings to the studies discussed above.[4-6]

Summary and Implications: In patients with RRMS, oral BG-12 has been shown to be an effective disease-modifying therapy compared with glatiramer acetate or placebo. This gives physicians and patients more options for MS treatments than the established injectable therapies.

CLINICAL CASE: ORAL BG-12 FOR RELAPSING MULTIPLE SCLEROSIS

Case History:
A 41-year-old woman was diagnosed with RRMS after she had an episode of optic neuritis. Her brain MRI demonstrated multiple nonenhancing periventricular and juxtacortical lesions, with an asymptomatic enhancing lesion in the cerebellum. She can recall in her distant past an episode of 3 days of left arm heaviness and numbness. Her neurologist wants to start her on a disease-modifying therapy, but she has a phobia of needles and refuses to self-inject. She is concerned that there are no other options for her. Based on the results of the DEFINE and CONFIRM trial, what should you tell her?

Suggested Answer:
The DEFINE and CONFIRM trials demonstrated safety and effectiveness of oral BG-12. There are many treatment options for multiple sclerosis, including injectable, oral, and intravenous agents. Dimethyl fumarate is a good option, and because she has a phobia of needles, an injectable therapy may be less desirable.

References

1. Fox RJ, Miller DH, Phillips JT, et al. Placebo-controlled phase 3 study of oral BG-12 or glatiramer in multiple sclerosis. *N Engl J Med*. 2012;367:1087–1097.
2. Gold R, Kappos L, Arnold DL, et al. Placebo-controlled phase 3 study of oral BG-12 for relapsing multiple sclerosis. N Engl J Med. 2012;367:1098–1107
3. Polman CH, Reingold SC, Barkhof F, et al. Ethics of placebo-controlled trials in multiple sclerosis: a reassessment. *Neurol*. 2008;70(13 Pt 2):1134–1140.
4. Kappos L, Gold R, Miller DH, et al. Efficacy and safety of oral fumarate in patients with relapsing-remitting multiple sclerosis: a multicentre, randomized, double-blind, placebo-controlled phase IIb study. *Lancet*. 2008;372(9648):1463–1472.
5. Havrdova E, Hutchinson M, Kurukulasuriya NC, et al. Oral BG-12 (dimethyl fumarate) for relapsing-remitting multiple sclerosis: a review of DEFINE and CONFIRM. Evaluation of: Gold R, Kappos L, Arnold D, et al. Placebo-controlled phase 3 study of oral BG-12 for relapsing multiple sclerosis. N Engl J Med 2012;367:1098–107; and Fox RJ, Miller DH, Phillips JT, et al. Placebo-controlled phase 3 study of oral BG-12 or glatiramer in multiple sclerosis. N Engl J Med 2012;367:1087–97. *Expert Opin Pharmacother*. 2013;14(15):2145–2156.
6. Bar-Or A, Gold R, Kappos L, et al. Clinical efficacy of BG-12 (dimethyl fumarate) in patients with relapsing-remitting multiple sclerosis: subgroup analyses of the DEFINE study. *J Neurol*. 2013;260(9):2297–2305.

SECTION VII

Neurocritical Care

Therapeutic Hypothermia for Cardiac Arrest, Part I
The HACA Trial

TEDDY S. YOUN

> Our results show that among patients in whom spontaneous circulation had been restored after cardiac arrest due to ventricular fibrillation, systemic cooling to a bladder temperature between 32°C and 34°C for 24 hours increased the chance of survival and of a favorable neurologic outcome..., as compared with standard normothermic life support.
> —THE HYPOTHERMIA AFTER CARDIAC ARREST (HACA) STUDY GROUP[1]

Research Question: Does moderate systemic hypothermia (e.g., 32°–34°C for 24 hours) increase rates of neurologic recovery after resuscitation from cardiac arrest due to ventricular fibrillation (VF)?[1]

Funding: Grants from the Biomedicine and Health Programme (BIOMED 2) implemented under the Fourth RTD Framework Programme 1994–1998 of the EU, the Austrian Ministry of Science and Transport, and the Austrian Science Foundation. Kinetic Concepts (Wareham, United Kingdom) provided the TheraKool cooling device.

Year Study Began: 1996

Year Study Published: 2002

Study Location: 9 participating sites in Austria, Belgium, Finland, Germany, and Italy

Who Was Studied: Patients aged 18–75 years who suffer a witnessed cardiac arrest (i.e., VF or pulseless ventricular tachycardia as the initial cardiac rhythm, from a presumed cardiac origin for the arrest). Only an estimated downtime of 5–15 minutes from the patient's witnessed collapse to the first attempt at resuscitation by emergency medical personnel, and an interval of no more than 60 minutes from collapse to return of spontaneous circulation (ROSC), were allowable for enrolled patients.

Who Was Excluded: Patients were excluded if they met any of the following criteria:

- A tympanic-membrane temperature <30°C on admission,
- A comatose state before the cardiac arrest due to drug administration that depressed the central nervous system,
- Pregnancy,
- Response to verbal commands after ROSC and before randomization,
- Sustained hypotension (mean arterial pressure <60 mm Hg) for >30 minutes after ROSC and before randomization,
- Sustained hypoxemia (arterial oxygen saturation <85%) for >15 minutes after ROSC and before randomization,
- A terminal illness that preceded the arrest,
- Factors that made participation in follow-up unlikely,
- Enrollment in another study,
- Occurrence of cardiac arrest after the arrival of emergency medical personnel, or
- Known preexisting coagulopathy.

How Many Patients Enrolled: 275

Study Overview: See Figure 18.1 for a summary of the study design.

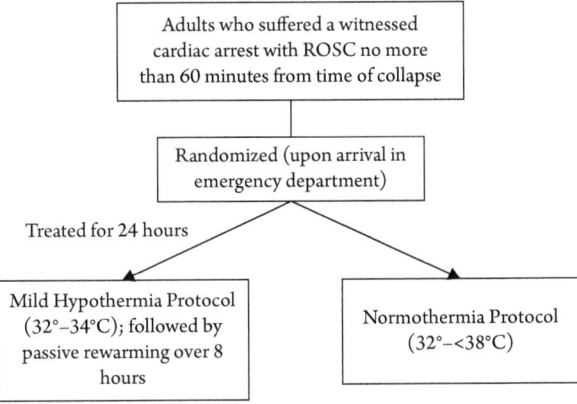

Figure 18.1 Summary of Study Design.

Study intervention:

- All patients: A temperature was taken on admission with an infrared tympanic thermometer. Further measurements were made from a bladder temperature probe that was placed with a Foley catheter during the study time period. All patients received sedation, analgesia, and a paralytic for 32 hours with intravenous administration of midazolam, fentanyl, and pancuronium, respectively.
- Mild hypothermia protocol: An external cooling device, consisting of a mattress with a cover that delivers cold air over the entire body, was used to reach the target bladder temperature range (32°–34°C) within 4 hours after ROSC. If this goal range was not met, ice packs were also used.
- Normothermia protocol: These patients received standard protocol-driven intensive care.

Follow-Up: Neurologic outcome within the first 6 months after arrest (See Table 18.1).

Table 18.1. CEREBRAL PERFORMANCE CATEGORIES (CPC) SCALE

CPC 1: Good cerebral performance: conscious, alert, able to work
CPC 2: Moderate cerebral disability: conscious, can carry out independent activities
CPC 3: Severe neurologic disability: conscious, dependent on others for daily support
CPC 4: Coma or vegetative state
CPC 5: Dead

Adapted from Jennett B, Bond M. Assessment of outcome after severe brain damage. *Lancet.* 1975;1(7905):480–484.

Endpoints: Primary outcome: Favorable neurologic outcome within six months after cardiac arrest, as measured by the Pittsburgh Cerebral-Performance Category (CPC) Scale as a CPC 1 or CPC 2 (See Table 18.1). Secondary outcomes: Mortality within 6 months and rates of complications within 7 days after cardiac arrest. Complications recorded included bleeding of any severity, pneumonia, sepsis, pancreatitis, renal failure, pulmonary edema, seizures, arrhythmias, and pressure sores.

RESULTS

- At 6 months, more patients in the hypothermia group had a favorable neurologic outcome versus the normothermia group (See Table 18.2).
- There was no significant difference in any of the tracked complications; however, an analysis of total complications favored a trend toward a higher rate of infection in the hypothermia group.

Table 18.2. SUMMARY OF NEUROLOGIC OUTCOME AND MORTALITY AT SIX MONTHS

Outcome	No./Total No. (%) Normothermia	Hypothermia	Risk Ratio (95% CI)	P Value
Favorable Neurologic Outcome	39	55	1.40 (1.08–1.81)	0.009
Death	55	41	0.74 (0.58–0.95)	0.02

Criticisms and Limitations: The criticisms of this study include the following. In its design, the study was only blinded to the study outcome assessors, but not to the treating attending physicians. The original investigators noted this was due to the design of the cooling device. Of note, more bystander CPR was performed in the normothermia group than the hypothermia group, which may speak to some confounding effect from bystander CPR on neurologic outcome. As well, in the initial characterization of the study group, little detail was given regarding the neurological examination findings of patients, specifically brainstem reflexes, prior to randomization, other than being comatose (personal communication). Therefore, it was unclear if the two groups were similar with regard to coma severity.

With regard to cooling, there were several limitations. The air mattress used for cooling in this trial was ineffective; 70% of patients also required ice packs to reach target temperature. The time to target cooling temperature also took on average 8 hours versus faster times in other comparative studies. As well, the normothermia group actually became hyperthermic on average, a variable not well controlled for in the study. This may have contributed to worse outcomes in this group.

Finally, due to the very strict inclusion and exclusion criteria, only 8% of the eligible patients were included in the trial. Questions over its generalizability to groups of patients with lower risk for brain damage and to those with cardiac arrest due to causes other than VF warrant further studies.

Other Relevant Studies and Information:

- Since the publication of this trial and the Australian trial in the following chapter,[1,2] several smaller studies on therapeutic hypothermia have been performed.[3,4]
- Recent randomized controlled trials have sought to refine two key variables with therapeutic hypothermia: target temperature ranges for therapeutic hypothermia and time to target temperature (with the use of pre-hospital versus in-hospital cooling protocols.
- Nielsen et al.[5] found that when comparing a targeted temperature range of 33°–36°C (i.e., prevention of fever), cooling to 33°C provided no additional benefit versus cooling to 36°C. This may suggest a permissive hypothermia range of 33°–36°C may be acceptable if clinicians feel uncomfortable cooling specific patients down to the lower range.
- Kim et al.[6] performed the largest blinded randomized controlled trial in therapeutic hypothermia to answer a focused question as to whether out-of-hospital initiation of therapeutic hypothermia by rapid infusion of cold saline confers any benefit to neurological outcome. They found that there was an increased risk for systemic complications associated with a rapid 2-liter infusion of cold saline (i.e., pulmonary edema and risk for cardiac rearrest) that outweighed any benefit in neurologic outcome or survival.

Summary and Implications: The HACA trial was one of two studies that demonstrated that active cooling for mild-to-moderate hypothermia improved the rate of favorable neurologic outcome and reduced mortality. In 2003, the International Liaison Committee on Resuscitation's Advanced Life Support Task Force[7] began recommending that (1) unconscious adult patients with spontaneous circulation after out-of-hospital cardiac arrest should be cooled to 32°–34°C for 12–24 hours when the initial rhythm was VF, and (2) such cooling may also be beneficial for other rhythms for patients experiencing an in-hospital cardiac arrest.

Especially in the context of the aforementioned more recent Nielsen et al. study,[6] further studies are necessary to determine the ideal method, duration, and range for therapeutic hypothermia in this patient population.

> **CLINICAL CASE: THERAPEUTIC HYPOTHERMIA FOR POST–CARDIAC ARREST**
>
> Please refer to the case at the end of Chapter 19.

References

1. Hypothermia after Cardiac Arrest Study G. Mild therapeutic hypothermia to improve the neurologic outcome after cardiac arrest. *N Engl J Med.* 2002;346: 549–556.
2. Bernard SA, Gray TW, Buist MD, et al. Treatment of comatose survivors of out-of-hospital cardiac arrest with induced hypothermia. *N Engl J Med.* 2002;346: 557–563.
3. Hachimi-Idrissi S, Corne L, Ebinger G, Michotte Y, Huyghens L. Mild hypothermia induced by a helmet device: a clinical feasibility study. *Resuscitation.* 2001;51:275–281.
4. Laurent I, Adrie C, Vinsonneau C, et al. High-volume hemofiltration after out-of-hospital cardiac arrest: a randomized study. *J Am Coll Cardiol.* 2005;46(3):432–437.
5. Nielsen N, Wetterslev J, Cronberg T, et al. Targeted temperature management at 33°C versus 36°C after cardiac arrest. *N Engl J Med.* 2013;369(23):2197–2206.
6. Kim F, Nichol G, Maynard C, et al. Effect of prehospital induction of mild hypothermia on survival and neurological status among adults with cardiac arrest. *JAMA.* 2014;311(1):45–52.
7. Nolan JP, Morley PT, Hoek TL, Hickey RW. Therapeutic hypothermia after cardiac arrest. An advisory statement by the Advanced Life Support Task Force of the International Liaison Committee on Resuscitation. *Resuscitation.* 2003;57: 231–235.

19

Therapeutic Hypothermia for Cardiac Arrest, Part II

The Australian Trial

TEDDY S. YOUN

> Our preliminary observations suggest that treatment with moderate hypothermia appears to improve outcomes in patients with coma after resuscitation from out-of-hospital arrest.
> —BERNARD ET AL.[1]

Research Question: Does moderate hypothermia (33°C) in patients who remain unconscious after resuscitation from out-of-hospital cardiac arrest within 2 hours after the return of spontaneous circulation improve neurologic outcome?[1]

Funding: None noted.

Year Study Began: 1996

Year Study Published: 2002

Study Location: Four participating hospitals (both in the emergency department and in intensive care units [ICU]) in Melbourne, Australia.

Who Was Studied: Patients with an initial cardiac rhythm of ventricular fibrillation (VF) at the time of arrival of the ambulance, successful return of spontaneous circulation (ROSC), persistent coma after ROSC, and transfer to 1 of 4 participating emergency departments.

Who Was Excluded: Patients aged <18 years (men) or <50 years (women, to exclude the possibility of pregnancy), patients who had cardiogenic shock (a systolic blood pressure <90 mm Hg despite epinephrine infusion), or possible causes of coma other than cardiac arrest (i.e., drug overdose, head trauma, or stroke). Patients were also excluded if an ICU bed was not available at the participating hospital.

How Many Patients: 77

Study Overview: See Figure 19.1 for a summary of the study design.

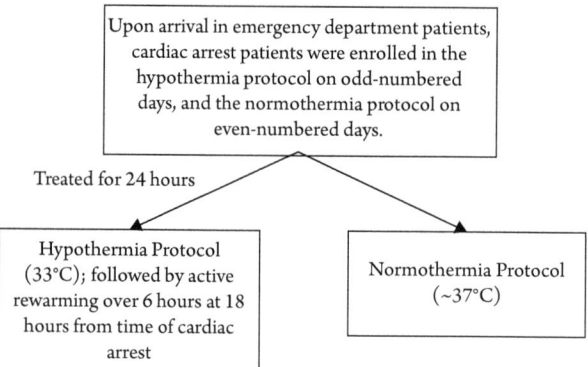

Figure 19.1 Summary of Study Design.

Study Intervention: Patients in the hypothermia group underwent vigorous cooling once in the emergency department with extensive application of ice packs around the head, neck, torso, and limbs until they reached a core temperature of 33°C. The patients were sedated and paralyzed with small doses of midazolam and vecuronium. At hour 18, they were actively rewarmed by external warming using a heated air blanket with continuous sedation and paralytic to suppress shivering. Patients assigned to normothermia were initially sedated and paralyzed; however, they did not receive any further dosing once they reached the target core temperature of 37°C. Passive rewarming was only used if there was mild spontaneous hypothermia.

Follow-Up: Assessment by a rehabilitation medicine specialist at the time of discharge from the hospital.

Endpoints: Primary outcomes: neurologic outcome at discharge from the hospital. Secondary outcomes: hemodynamic/physiological, biochemical, hematologic values of hypothermia.

RESULTS

- At the time of discharge, 21 of 43 patients in the hypothermia group (49%) were considered to have a good outcome (discharge to home or to a rehabilitation facility), versus 9 of 34 patients in the normothermia group (26%), $P = 0.046$, 95% confidence interval (CI), 13%–43% (see Table 19.1).
- The unadjusted odds ratio for a good outcome in the hypothermia group as compared with the normothermia group was 2.65 (95% CI range, 1.02–6.88; $P = 0.046$). After adjustment for baseline differences in age and time from collapse to return of spontaneous circulation, the odds ratio improved to 5.25 (95% CI range, 1.47–18.76; $P = 0.011$).
- There was no difference in the frequency of adverse events.
- There was no significant difference in hemodynamic, biochemical, or hematological values between the two arms, except for a lower cardiac index and hyperglycemia.

Table 19.1. OUTCOME OF PATIENTS AT DISCHARGE FROM THE HOSPITAL

Outcome	Hypothermia % (n = 43)	Normothermia % (n = 34)
Normal or minimal disability (able to care for self, discharged to home)	34.9	20.6
Moderate disability (discharged to a rehabilitation facility)	14.0	6.0
Severe disability, awake but completely dependent (discharged to a long-term nursing facility)	0	2.9
Severe disability, unconscious (discharged to a long-term nursing facility)	0	2.9
Death	51.2	67.6

Criticisms and Limitations: For this study, several limitations existed. First, it was a much smaller sample size than the HACA trial.[2] The definition of coma for the study was never defined. Interestingly, the study was not a true randomization. Instead, study coordinators enrolled patients to the hypothermia protocol on odd-numbered days and the normothermia protocol on even-numbered days, leading to the uneven number of patients in each arm. Finally, the patients were actively rewarmed, which can lead to hypotension and cerebral edema. However, this would have led to worse outcomes in the hypothermia group, if anything.

Other Relevant Studies and Information:

- Since the publication of this trial and the HACA trial outlined in Chapter 18,[1,2] several smaller studies on therapeutic hypothermia have been performed.[3,4]
- Recent randomized controlled trials have sought to refine two key variables with therapeutic hypothermia: target temperature ranges for therapeutic hypothermia and time to target temperature (with the use of pre-hospital versus in-hospital cooling protocols.
- Nielsen et al.[5] found that when comparing a targeted temperature range of 33°–36°C (i.e., prevention of fever), cooling to 33°C provided no additional benefit versus cooling to 36°C. This may suggest a permissive hypothermia range of 33°–36°C may be acceptable if clinicians feel uncomfortable cooling specific patients down to the lower range.
- Kim et al.[6] performed the largest blinded randomized controlled trial in therapeutic hypothermia to answer a focused question as to whether out-of-hospital initiation of therapeutic hypothermia by rapid infusion of cold saline confers any benefit to neurological outcome. They found that there was an increased risk for systemic complications associated with a rapid 2-liter infusion of cold saline (i.e., pulmonary edema and risk for cardiac rearrest) that outweighed any benefit in neurologic outcome or survival.

Summary and Implications: The Australian trial was one of two studies that demonstrated that active cooling for mild-to-moderate hypothermia improved the rate of favorable neurologic outcome and reduced mortality. In 2003, the International Liaison Committee on Resuscitation's Advanced Life Support Task Force[7] began recommending that (1) unconscious adult patients with spontaneous circulation after out-of-hospital cardiac arrest should be cooled to 32°–34°C for 12–24 hours when the initial rhythm was VF, and (2) such cooling may also be beneficial for other rhythms for patients experiencing an in-hospital cardiac arrest.

Especially in the context of the aforementioned more recent Nielsen et al. study,[5] further studies are necessary to determine the ideal method, duration, and range for therapeutic hypothermia in this patient population.

CLINICAL CASE: THERAPEUTIC HYPOTHERMIA FOR POST–CARDIAC ARREST

Case History:
A 45-year-old male carpenter is rushed to the emergency department by ambulance after his wife sees him outside on the ground clutching his chest 5 minutes after he was last seen normal moving wood outside the house. She immediately performs cardiopulmonary resuscitation when she finds him on the ground unconscious. She asks her daughter to call 911. Paramedics arrive within 20 minutes from the time of arrest and find that he is in VF. A return of spontaneous circulation occurs after 1 dose of epinephrine and administration of 300 J of direct current shock.

The paramedics arrive within 30 minutes of the time of arrest to the emergency department. On examination, the patient's vital signs are stable and a pulse is palpable. The patient has a temperature of 37°C on admission. Neurologically, the patient is comatose, and has decorticate posturing to noxious stimuli, but all brainstem reflexes are intact.

Based on the results of the HACA and Australian trials, should this patient undergo therapeutic hypothermia?

Suggested Answer:
Both the HACA and Australian trials established that cooling this patient to a range of 32°–34°C for 12–24 hours will improve survival or neurological outcome by 14%–23%. The ideal method of cooling is still unknown, but could include surface cooling versus more invasive vascular methods. Especially in the context of the aforementioned more recent Nielsen et al. study,[5] further studies are necessary to determine the ideal method, duration, and range for therapeutic hypothermia in this patient population.

References

1. Bernard SA, Gray TW, Buist MD, et al. Treatment of comatose survivors of out-of-hospital cardiac arrest with induced hypothermia. *N Engl J Med.* 2002;346:557–563.
2. Hypothermia after Cardiac Arrest Study G. Mild therapeutic hypothermia to improve the neurologic outcome after cardiac arrest. *N Engl J Med.* 2002;346:549–556.
3. Hachimi-Idrissi S, Corne L, Ebinger G, Michotte Y, Huyghens L. Mild hypothermia induced by a helmet device: a clinical feasibility study. *Resuscitation.* 2001;51:275–281.
4. Laurent I, Adrie C, Vinsonneau C, et al. High-volume hemofiltration after out-of-hospital cardiac arrest: a randomized study. *J Am Coll Cardiol.* 2005;46(3):432–437.
5. Nielsen N, Wetterslev J, Cronberg T, et al. Targeted temperature management at 33°C versus 36°C after cardiac arrest. *N Engl J Med.* 2013;369(23):2197–2206.
6. Kim F, Nichol G, Maynard C, et al. Effect of prehospital induction of mild hypothermia on survival and neurological status among adults with cardiac arrest. *JAMA.* 2014;311(1):45–52.
7. Nolan JP, Morley PT, Hoek TL, Hickey RW. Therapeutic hypothermia after cardiac arrest: an advisory statement by the Advanced Life Support Task Force of the International Liaison Committee on Resuscitation. *Resuscitation.* 2003;57:231–235.

Decompressive Craniectomy for Diffuse Traumatic Brain Injury
The DECRA Trial

SHIVANI GHOSHAL

> Among adults with severe diffuse traumatic brain injury and refractory intracranial hypertension in the ICU . . . patients in the craniectomy group had a lower median score on the Extended Glasgow Outcome Scale and a higher risk of an unfavorable outcome than patients receiving standard [medical] care.
>
> —COOPER ET AL.[1]

Research Question: Is decompressive craniectomy or medical management more effective for obtaining better outcomes in traumatic brain injury (TBI) patients with increased intracranial pressure (ICP) after receiving "first-tier" therapies?[1]

Funding: National Health and Medical Research Council of Australia.

Year Study Began: 2002

Year Study Published: 2011

Study Location: 15 hospitals in Australia, New Zealand, and Saudi Arabia.

Who Was Studied: TBI patients aged <60 years with (1) an initial Glasgow Coma Scale (GCS) score of <9 and (2) elevated intracranial pressure of >20 mm Hg despite medical therapy for >15 minutes in 1 hour.

Who Was Excluded: Patients with bilateral dilated unreactive pupils, with surgically removable intracranial mass lesions, with spinal cord injury or cardiac arrest at the scene of injury.

How Many Patients: 155

Study Overview: See Table 20.1 for a summary of the study design.

Table 20.1. SUMMARY OF STUDY DESIGN

Condition	Randomized Patients Allocated (N = 155)
Early decompressive craniectomy	73
Standard medical management	82

Study Intervention: All patients initially received "first-tier" interventions for elevations in ICP, including optimized sedation, $PaCO_2$ management, osmotic therapy, pharmacological paralysis, and external ventricular drainage. Patients randomized to the decompressive craniectomy trial arm received bifronto-temporo-parietal decompressive craniectomy with bilateral dural openings to maximize ICP reduction. Patients randomized to standard medical management received further medical interventions drawn from the Brain Trauma Foundation Clinical Practice Guidelines,[2] including mild hypothermia (to 35°C) and barbiturate infusions.

Follow-Up: 6 months.

Endpoints: Primary outcome: difference in the Glasgow Outcome Score - Extended (GOSE) between groups using ordinal logistic regression analysis at 6 months (see Table 20.2). Secondary outcomes: proportion of favorable outcomes (GOSE scores 5–8), mortality at 6 months, intracranial pressure following randomization, and number of days in the ICU and hospital.

RESULTS

- Table 20.3 summarizes functional outcomes in the study. At baseline, although patients with dilated unreactive pupils were excluded, the number of patients with bilateral (small) unreactive pupils—a

clinical indicator for more severe injury—was significantly higher in the decompressive craniectomy arm (27%) versus the medical management arm (12%).
  - After the primary outcome results were adjusted for 4 predetermined covariates, the differences in the 6-month primary outcome remained significant; after they were adjusted for the pupillary reactivity covariate alone, this difference was not significant.
- Four patients from the standard medical therapy group received decompressive craniectomies <72 hours after randomization due to clinical concerns from their care teams, and 15 patients (18%) from the standard medical therapy group underwent craniectomy >72 hours after randomization.
- After randomization, mean ICP was significantly lower in the decompressive craniectomy group (14.4 vs. 19.1 mm Hg, $P < 0.001$)
- Patients in the craniectomy group had significantly shorter durations of mechanical ventilation (11 vs. 15 days, $P < 0.001$) and ICU stay (13 vs. 18 days, $P < 0.001$), though the two groups showed no significant difference in total hospital days.
- Rates of death at 6-month follow up were similar between the craniectomy and standard medical groups —19% and 18%, respectively.

Table 20.2. EXTENDED GLASGOW OUTCOME SCALE

Score	Description
1—Dead	
2—Vegetative state	Unawareness with only reflex responses, periods of spontaneous eye opening
3—Low severe disability	Patient is dependent for daily support for mental or physical disability. Patient cannot be left alone for >8 hours
4—Upper severe disability	Patient is dependent for daily support for mental or physical disability. Patient cannot be left alone for >4 hours
5—Low moderate disability	Patients have some disability; they are independent at home but dependent otherwise. Patients at this level cannot return to work even with special arrangement.
6—Upper moderate disability	Patients have some disability; they are independent at home but dependent otherwise. Patients at this level may be able to return to work.
7—Low good recovery	Resumption of normal life, with capacity to work. Patient may have minor but disabling neurological or psychological deficits.
8—Upper good recovery	Resumption of normal life, with capacity to work. Patient may have minor but not disabling neurological or psychological deficits.

Table 20.3. SUMMARY OF DECRA'S KEY FINDINGS

Outcome	Decompressive Craniectomy	Medical Management	P Value
Median GOSE at 6 months	3	4	0.03
Poor functional outcome at 6 months (GOSE 1–4)	70%	51%	0.02

Criticisms and Limitations: The results of the study do not apply to TBI patients with mass lesions necessitating evacuation, nor to late (salvage) craniectomy. At baseline, the craniectomy group had significantly more patients with bilateral (small) nonreactive pupils. No other measure of injury severity was significantly different between the groups. For ethical reasons, there was crossover (19%) from the medical therapy group to eventual decompression, but nevertheless, craniectomy effectively decreased ICP.

Other Relevant Studies and Information:

- The completed RESCUE-ICP (Randomized Evaluation of Surgery with Craniectomy for Uncontrollable Elevation of Surgery with Craniectomy)[3] trial aims to further assess the impact of decompressive craniectomy for TBI patients with both diffuse injury and mass lesions, and with refractory increased ICP. RESCUE-ICP will further interpret results based on severity of individual patient characteristics. The study completed enrollment of 400 patients in 2014 and is awaiting analysis with 6-month follow-up data.
- The Brain Trauma Foundation supports medical management of severe TBI without mass lesions; the guidelines were last updated in 2007.[2] There are no current guidelines for appropriate use of craniectomy in this patient population.

Summary and Implications: For severe TBI patients without mass lesions, decompressive craniectomy for refractory ICP elevations after first-tier therapy was found to significantly lower ICP, reduce the number of days of mechanical ventilation, and reduce ICU length of stay. However, if the goal of therapy is to optimize the patient's functional outcome, the DECRA trial showed that decompressive craniectomy led to significantly worse 6-month functional outcomes versus third-tier medical therapies.

CLINICAL CASE: DECOMPRESSIVE CRANIECTOMY VERSUS MEDICAL MANAGEMENT FOR DIFFUSE TBI WITH INCREASED ICP

Case History:

A 27-year-old man presents as a motor vehicle crash victim. On initial assessment, he has a GCS score of 6. His CT scan shows no surgically removable mass lesions. Due to his poor exam and concern for cerebral edema after his injury, he receives ICP monitoring. Despite heavy optimized sedation, maintaining a $PaCO_2$ between 35 and 40, receiving repeated osmotic therapy, and undergoing external ventricular drainage, the patient still has an ICP >30 for 15 minutes within an hour. Based on the results of DECRA, how should this patient be treated to optimize his end functional outcome?

Suggested Answer:

In DECRA, decompressive craniectomy was found to more effectively lower refractory ICP and decrease the number of days in the ICU compared to second-tier medical therapy with barbiturate infusions and mild hypothermia. However, if the goal of therapy is to optimize the patient's functional outcome, DECRA showed decompressive craniectomy led to significantly worse 6-month functional outcomes in comparison to third-tier medical therapies. The study has limitations, including the study definition of refractory ICP and nonstandardized rehabilitation. In this case, medical therapy with barbiturate infusion and mild hypothermia may control ICP sufficiently and lead to a better functional outcome in the long term. The upcoming RESCUE-ICP trial results may help guide clinical practice further.

References

1. The DECRA Investigators. Decompressive craniectomy in diffuse traumatic brain injury. *N Engl J Med*. 2011;364(16):1493–1502.
2. Guidelines for the management of severe traumatic brain injury. *Journal of Neurotrauma*; 2007:24 (Supplement 1).
3. Hutchinson PJ, Kirkpatrick PJ. RESCUEicp Central Study Team: craniectomy in diffuse traumatic brain injury. *N Engl J Med*. 2011;365:375.

21
Nimodipine for Subarachnoid Hemorrhage

TEDDY S. YOUN

> [T]his study suggests that patients who are essentially neurologically normal after a subarachnoid hemorrhage from an aneurysm will benefit from oral administration of nimodipine for three weeks after the hemorrhage.
> —ALLEN ET AL.[1]

Research Question: Does a calcium channel antagonist, like nimodipine, prevent or alter the severity of ischemic neurologic deficits due to vasospasm in patients who survive the initial subarachnoid hemorrhage from an intracranial aneurysm?[1]

Funding: Miles Pharmaceuticals (West Haven, Connecticut).

Year Study Began: 1979

Year Study Published: 1982

Study Location: Five university centers in the United States.

Who Was Studied: Patients aged 15–80 years who had an aneurysmal subarachnoid hemorrhage within 96 hours from time of enrollment and was treated by surgical clipping; who had normal results on a neurologic examination performed just before the start of medication, which could include the following findings: a stiff neck, headache, fever, or photophobia; drowsiness but with orientation at least to person, city, and year; or the presence of isolated cranial-nerve palsies. Before enrollment, everyone was evaluated by head CT scan, documentation of a subarachnoid hemorrhage by either CT scan or cerebrospinal fluid examination, and demonstration of an intracranial aneurysm by angiography.

Who Was Excluded: The following types of patients were excluded:

- Patients without evidence of a subarachnoid hemorrhage by radiographic findings or by cerebrospinal fluid examination.
- Patients in whom the etiology of subarachnoid hemorrhage was not an intracranial aneurysm.
- Patients who did not receive intracranial surgery within 14 days of entry into the study (unless a neurologic deficit or some other medical problem made surgery inadvisable).
- Patients who had moderate to severe neurologic deficits on entry (e.g., Hunt & Hess Scale Grade ≥3).

How Many Patients: 116

Study Overview: See Figure 21.1 for a summary of the study design.

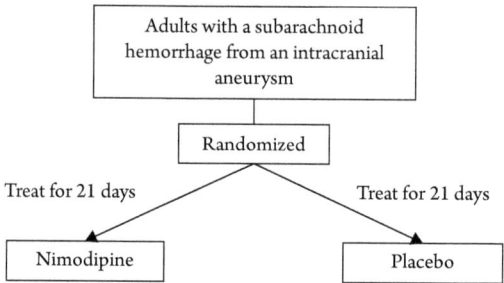

Figure 21.1 Summary of the Study's Design.

Study Intervention: Patients in the nimodipine group received 0.7 mg/kg (adjusted to the nearest full 10 mg capsule) of nimodipine orally (by capsule or liquid) as an initial dose, followed by 0.35 mg/kg every 4 hours for 21 days. Patients in the placebo group received an oral placebo.

Follow-Up: Neurologic status at the end of 21-day treatment period (see Table 21.1)

Table 21.1. CLASSIFICATION OF NEUROLOGIC OUTCOMES
AFTER 21 DAYS OF TREATMENT[a]

Normal	Neurologically intact, except 4/5 strength may be present in 1 extremity only.
Mild/moderate	A patient must have a neurologic deficit that does not meet the definition of "severe."
Severe	One or more of the following: 1. Eye Opening: None, or only in response to pain. 2. Verbal Response: None, or incomprehensible sounds. 3. Complete lack of orientation. 4. Motor response: None, or withdrawal/posturing in response to pain. 5. Motor strength: Weakness in more than one extremity, with 2/5 or less strength in one of the extremities.

[a] Adapted from Table 1 of Allen GS, Ahn HS, Preziosi TJ. Cerebral arterial spasm—a controlled trial of nimodipine in patients with subarachnoid hemorrhage. *N Engl J Med.* 1983;308:620.

Endpoints: Primary outcomes: the development of a neurologic deficit from cerebral arterial spasm and the severity of the deficit at the end of the treatment period. Secondary outcomes: mean values for the greatest degree of spasm on angiogram; unenhanced, pre-entry head CT-scan rankings; head CT scans of patients with deficits from spasm that were ranked by amount of blood in the basal subarachnoid spaces.

RESULTS

- After 21 days of treatment, more patients in the placebo (8) versus nimodipine group (1) had severe neurologic deficits from cerebral arterial spasm, with a relative risk reduction of 86% (see Table 21.2). A significant benefit was not seen when the whole population was considered.
- There was no significant difference in the incidence or severity of angiographic vasospasm between the two arms.
- Adverse effects from the intervention were not noted in this study. Oral nimodipine did not increase rates of rebleeding or surgical complications.
- Interestingly, the investigators found that a large amount of basal subarachnoid hemorrhage did not negatively impact the effect of nimodipine.

- In the placebo arm, the severity of the neurologic deficits from spasm correlated with more blood in the basal subarachnoid spaces on their initial CT scans and with the severity of their spasm at the onset of deficits ($P < 0.05$).

Table 21.2. SUMMARY OF NEUROLOGIC OUTCOMES[a]

Outcome	Placebo (n = 60)	Nimodipine (n = 56)
No neurologic deficits from any cause	28	24
Neurologic deficits from cause other than vasospasm	16	19
Neurologic deficits from spasm, according to neurologic outcome		
Normal	6	8
Mild-moderate	2 (1 mild disorientation, 1 mild weakness)	4 (1 mild disorientation, 2 mild weakness, 1 w/ disorientation, mild weakness, and mild aphasia)
Severe	8 (3 deaths, 1 coma, 4 severe neurologic deficits)	1 (1 death)

[a] Adapted from Table 3 of Allen GS, Ahn HS, Preziosi TJ. Cerebral arterial spasm—a controlled trial of nimodipine in patients with subarachnoid hemorrhage. *N Engl J Med*. 1983;308:620.

Criticisms and Limitations: There were several limitations in this study. First, it had a small sample size. Also, since the study did not have a treatment crossover model, there may have been unknown factors that may have been not normally distributed between the two treatment arms. The dose of nimodipine was effective, but not maximal in this study. Due to concerns for its safety profile in humans, a dose-response or dose-toxicity curve was not trialed in this study.

With regards to the patient selection, patients were required to be normal (or near normal) in this study; thus, it is unclear whether nimodipine is effective in patients with higher clinical grades. Patients with Fisher scale scores of 1 and 4 were included in this study, and these patients have a low incidence of vasospasm. Aneurysms were treated late in this trial, and the rebleeding rate was high, which is known to lead to worse outcomes and a higher rate of vasospasm.

Finally, with regard to treatment side effects, nimodipine, like all calcium channel blockers, is known to cause hypotension. However, systemic hypotension as a significant event was not reported in this trial. Several of the morbidities in this trial occurred secondary to surgical clipping or rebleeding, and thus were unrelated to vasospasm.

Other Relevant Studies and Information:

- Prior to this trial, Dr. Allen and colleagues showed that the source of calcium (which is necessary with ATP for smooth muscle contraction) is extracellular for brain arteries instead of intracellular for systemic arteries.[2] This study suggested that, ideally, a drug that inhibited the flow of calcium into the intracranial arterial smooth muscle cells would prevent arterial contraction without producing severe systemic hypotension.
- In follow-up, Dr. Allen and colleagues then performed in vivo studies in a subarachnoid hemorrhage model in dogs that demonstrated that nimodipine, a calcium channel antagonist, prevented angiographic spasm without systemic hypotension.[3]
- Immediately following this trial, the British Aneurysm Nimodipine Trial (BRANT)[4] looked at a larger group of 554 patients recruited during a 3-year span from 4 British neurosurgical units. This trial demonstrated that oral nimodipine, at 60 mg given every 4 hours, was well-tolerated and reduced cerebral infarction from 33% to 22% on CT scans. Additionally, poor outcomes were reduced to 20% in the treated group versus 33% in the placebo-group. The study also noted mild reductions in blood pressure with nimodipine, but reported no adverse effects.
- Many studies since Allen's original paper have looked into use of different calcium antagonists and different formulations of nimodipine. A Cochrane analysis of 7 clinical trials found that nimodipine reduces poor outcome by approximately 50% when given orally; however, there is no evidence currently to suggest that intravenous administration of nimodipine impacts outcome.[5]
- The current recommendations from the Neurocritical Care Society on the critical care management of aneurysmal subarachnoid hemorrhage suggest oral nimodipine 60 milligrams every 4 hours should be given for a period of 21 days from symptom onset. If that dosing schedule results in hypotension, then dosing intervals should be changed to more frequent lower doses. If hypotension continues to occur, then nimodipine may be discontinued.[6]

Summary and Implications: This double-blind randomized controlled trial established that oral nimodipine is a part of standard treatment for aneurysmal subarachnoid hemorrhage, which helps reduce the rate of severe neurologic deficits related to vasospasm.

CLINICAL CASE: NIMODIPINE FOR SUBARACHNOID HEMORRHAGE

Case History:
A 65-year-old right-handed woman with a past medical history of hypertension and prior smoking is rushed to the emergency department by ambulance after her daughter found her unconscious after a syncopal episode while outside shoveling snow. She was unconscious for approximately 3–5 minutes. En route to the outside hospital, she becomes progressively more alert, and on arrival to the hospital, her neurologic examination is fully intact except for some mild neck stiffness and headache.

A noncontrast head computed tomography (CT) scan shows extensive subarachnoid hemorrhage filling the basilar cisterns and sylvian fissure on the right. A CT angiogram reveals a right posterior communicating artery aneurysm, 8 mm × 10 mm × 12 mm. This aneurysm is secured by endovascular coiling within the next 24 hours.

Based on the results of the Nimodipine after Subarachnoid Hemorrhage Study, should you give this patient nimodipine?

Suggested Answer:
The Nimodipine after Subarachnoid Hemorrhage trial established that oral nimodipine does not completely prevent the occurrence of neurologic ischemic deficits secondary to vasospasm, but that it does significantly reduce the rate of severe neurologic deficits, including death from vasospasm alone.

Thus, she should receive nimodipine 60 mg every 4 hours orally, either in capsule or liquid form, and it should be administered for a 21-day period from the time of onset for her subarachnoid hemorrhage. This can be clinically modified to a dose of 30 mg every 2 hours if she develops systemic hypotension from the 60 mg dose.

References

1. Allen GS, Ahn HS, Preziosi TJ, et al. Cerebral arterial spasm—a controlled trial of nimodipine in patients with subarachnoid hemorrhage. *N Engl J Med.* 1983; 308:619–624.
2. Allen GS, Gross CJ, Henderson LM, et al. Cerebral arterial spasm. Part 4. In vitro effects of temperature, serotonin analogues, large non-physioloigcal concentrations of serotonin, and extracellular calcium and magnesium on serotonin-induced contractions of the canine basilar artery. *J Neurosurg.* 1976;44:585–593.
3. Cohen RJ, Allen GS. Cerebral arterial spasm: the role of calcium in vitro and in vivo analysis of treatment with nifedipine and nimodipine. In: Wilkins RH, ed. *Cerebral Arterial Spasm.* Baltimore: Williams and Wilkins; 1979:527–532.
4. Pickard JD, Murray GD, Illingworth R, et al. Effect of oral nimodipine on cerebral infarction and outcome after subarachnoid hemorrhage: British aneurysm nimodipine trial. *BMJ.* 1989;298:636–642.
5. Dorhout MS, Rinkel GJ, Feigin VL, et al. Calcium antagonists for aneurysmal subarachnoid hemorrhage. *Cochrane Database Syst Rev.* 2008;(4):CD000277
6. Diringer MN, Bleck TP, Hemphill JC III, et al. Critical care management of patients following aneurysmal subarachnoid hemorrhage: recommendations from the Neurocritical Care Society's Multidisciplinary Consensus Conference. *Neurocrit Care.* 2011:15(2):211–240.

SECTION VIII

Neuromuscular Disease

22

IVIG versus Plasma Exchange for Guillain-Barré Syndrome

IRENE HWA YANG

> In treatment of severe Guillain-Barré syndrome ... plasma exchange and intravenous immunoglobulin had equivalent efficacy. The combination of plasma exchange with intravenous immunoglobulin did not confer a significant advantage.
> —PLASMA EXCHANGE/SANDOGLOBULIN GUILLAIN-BARRÉ SYNDROME TRIAL GROUP[1]

Research Questions: Is intravenous immunoglobulin (IVIG) equally effective as or superior to plasma exchange (PE) as monotherapy for the treatment of Guillain-Barré syndrome? Is the combination of PE followed by IVIG superior to monotherapy alone?[1]

Funding: Sandoz AG (now part of Novartis AG), a pharmaceutical company.

Year Study Began: 1993

Year Study Published: 1997

Study Location: 38 centers in 11 countries.

Who Was Studied: Patients >16 years old who had the onset of neuropathic symptoms within the previous 14 days and who met accepted clinical and cerebrospinal fluid diagnostic criteria for Guillain-Barré syndrome as diagnosed by a qualified neurologist. In addition, patients had to have severe disease, defined by requiring assistance or being unable to walk, or requiring ventilatory support.

Who Was Excluded: Patients with atypical forms of Guillain-Barré syndrome including the Miller Fisher variant; those with other serious preexisting disease; and those with contraindications to receiving plasma exchange or IVIG were excluded.

How Many Patients: 379

Study Overview: See Figure 22.1 for a summary of the trial's design.

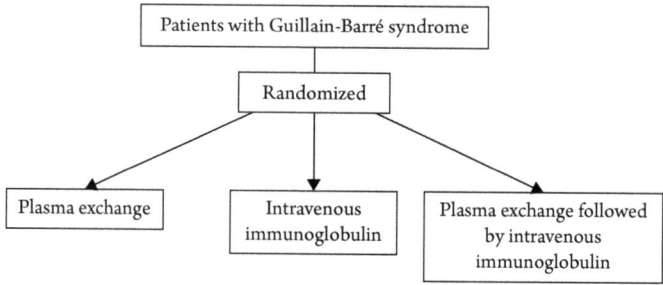

Figure 22.1: Summary of Study's Design.

Study Intervention: Patients in the plasma exchange group received five 50 mL/kg exchanges, which were completed on days 8–13 following randomization. In some cases, a sixth exchange was given to achieve a total exchange volume goal of 250 mL/kg.

Patients in the IVIG group received 0.4 g/kg of human IVIG (Sandoglobulin®) daily for a total of 5 days beginning on day 1 of randomization.

Patients in the plasma exchange plus IVIG group received five 50 mL/kg plasma exchanges starting on day 1 of randomization. This was followed by IVIG (Sandoglobulin®) dosed at 0.4 g/kg daily for 5 days starting on the day following the last plasma exchange.

Concurrent corticosteroid treatment for Guillain-Barré syndrome was discouraged. In some patients, repeating treatment with the original randomized treatment was permitted in the case of relapse. Relapse was defined as an increase of 1 or more on disability grade scoring for at least 1 week after the grade had been stable or had improved by ≥1 for at least a week (see Table 22.1).

Table 22.1. DISABILITY GRADES

Score	Description
0	• "Healthy, no signs or symptoms of Guillain-Barré syndrome"
1	• "Minor signs or symptoms and able to run"
2	• "Able to walk 5 m across an open space without assistance"
3	• "Able to walk 5 m across an open space with the help of one person and waist-level walking frame, stick, or sticks"
4	• "Chairbound/bedbound; unable to walk"
5	• "Requiring assisted ventilation"
6	• "Dead"

Follow-Up: 48 weeks.

Endpoints: Primary outcome was assessed by disability grade, arm grade, and vital capacity at randomization and at 2, 4, 8, 12, 24, and 48 weeks (see Table 22.2). Secondary outcomes were time from randomization to unaided walking, time to ventilator independence, and average rate of recovery based on disability grade over 48 weeks. Other outcomes included mortality and the fraction of patients with disability grade 3 or higher at 48 weeks.

Table 22.2. ARM GRADES

Score	Description
0	• "Normal"
1	• "Minor signs or symptoms but able to put hand on top of head when sitting with head upright, and able to oppose thumb to each fingertip"
2	• "Able to do either task in 1, but not both"
3	• "Some movements but unable to perform either of the tasks in 2"
4	• "No movement"
5	• "Dead"

RESULTS

- There were no significant differences between the three treatment groups with respect to mean disability grade improvement after 4 weeks, or on the time to walk unaided (see Table 22.3).
- Although not significant, the time to unaided walking was slightly shorter in the PE+IVIG group compared to PE or IVIG alone.
- 12% of patients who required ventilation died, compared to 1.7% of patients who did not need ventilation.
- Complications because of treatment occurred in 8 patients in the PE group, 6 patients in the IVIG group, and 15 patients in the PE+IVIG group.

- 13.8% of PE patients received less than 75% of the planned dose, compared to 2.3% of IVIG patients.
- Following 48 weeks, relapses occurred in 7 patients in the PE group, 4 in the IVIG group, and 9 in the PE+IVIG group.

Table 22.3. SUMMARY OF THE TRIAL'S KEY FINDINGS

Outcome	PE Group	IVIG Group	PE + IVIG Group
Mean change in disability grade after 4 weeks	0.9	0.8	1.1
Median days to stop artificial ventilation	29	26	18
Median days to unaided walking	49	51	40
Number of patients unable to walk unaided after 48 weeks	19 (16.7%)	21 (16.5%)	17 (13.7%)
Deaths	5 (4.1%)	6 (4.6%)	8 (8.3%)

Criticisms and Limitations: There was no true control group in the study so it is unclear whether any of the treatments were superior to supportive care alone.

Although similarly efficacious, a larger percentage of plasma exchange patients received <75% of the planned dose compared to IVIG patients, primarily because of side effects and complications. This demonstrates the challenges that can occur in receiving plasma exchange therapy. It may be difficult to distinguish between the complications of Guillain-Barré syndrome and the side effects of treatment in the study. However, these determinations were performed by a large number of experienced physicians across several countries and centers.

Other Relevant Studies and Information:

- Plasma exchange therapy has been shown elsewhere to be effective in patients with severe Guillain-Barré syndrome when compared to no exchange.[2,3]
- Other studies have also shown that IVIG is at least as effective as plasma exchange therapy.[4,5]
- Guidelines from the American Academy of Neurology conclude that plasma exchange or IVIG hastens recovery and should be used as disease-modifying treatments in patients with Guillain-Barré syndrome.[6] Based on the information in the literature, the European Federation of Neurological Societies recommends IVIG or plasma exchange as first-line treatment for Guillain-Barré syndrome, with IVIG being more favorable given the side effect profile.[7]
- Treatments of plasma exchange followed immediately by IVIG is not recommended.[6]

Summary and Implications: In patients with Guillain-Barré syndrome, treatment with plasma exchange or IVIG is equally efficacious. Combination treatment of plasma exchange immediately followed by IVIG has not been established as superior to monotherapy. There is an ongoing study to determine if two doses of IVIG are better than a single dose in those still severely affected by Guillain-Barré syndrome 2 weeks after the first dose of IVIG.

CLINICAL CASE: TREATMENT OF GUILLAIN-BARRÉ SYNDROME

Case History:

A 52-year-old man complains of a 2-week history of progressive weakness. He has no past medical history and has been in his usual state of health except for a gastrointestinal illness 2 weeks prior. Since that time, he has noticed weakness of his legs, which over the past few days has involved his arms and hands as well. He is now unable to walk without assistance from his wife because of his leg weakness. He also complains of mild tingling in his feet.

On examination, the patient's vital signs are unremarkable. He has severe symmetric weakness of his legs and mild weakness of his hands. Sensory exam is notable for diminished vibration and light touch sensation in his feet. Reflexes are diminished bilaterally, with absent plantar and Achilles reflexes.

A lumbar puncture reveals a CSF protein of 123 mg/dL. CSF cell count is <5 cells/mm^3 and CSF glucose is 65 mg/dL.

Based on the results of this trial, how should this patient be treated?

Suggested Answer:

Based on the information presented, this patient has Guillain-Barré syndrome. Features consistent with the diagnosis of Guillain-Barré syndrome include preceding illness, progressive weakness in more than one limb, areflexia/hyporeflexia, mild sensory symptoms, and an elevated CSF protein with a cell count <10/mm^3.[8]

He should be treated with either plasma exchange or IVIG. There is no role for initial dual therapy with plasma exchange followed by IVIG as this does not improve outcome. Tailoring appropriate therapy depends on several factors including local hospital capabilities, risk factors, and patient preference. Plasma exchange may necessitate a need for central venous access, which can lead to further complications.[9] This patient should also be provided with supportive care including, but not limited to, ICU monitoring, ventilator support, and pain control as needed.

References

1. Randomised trial of plasma exchange, intravenous immunoglobulin, and combined treatments in Guillain-Barré syndrome. Plasma exchange/Sandoglobulin Guillain-Barré Syndrome Trial Group. *Lancet*. 1997;349:225–230.
2. Plasmapheresis and acute Guillain-Barré syndrome. The Guillain-Barré Syndrome Study Group. *Neurology*. 1985;35(9):1096.
3. Efficiency of plasma exchange in Guillain-Barré syndrome: role of replacement fluids. French Cooperative Group on Plasma Exchange in Guillain-Barré syndrome. *Ann Neurol*. 1987;22(6):753.
4. FGA van der Meché, Schmitz PI. A randomized trial comparing intravenous immune globulin and plasma exchange in Guillain-Barré syndrome. *NEJM*. 1992;326:1123–1129.
5. Bril V, Ilse WK, Pearce R, Dhanani A, Sutton D, Kong K. Pilot trial of immunoglobulin versus plasma exchange in patients with Guillain-Barré syndrome. *Neurology*. 1996;46:100–103.
6. Hughes RA, Wijdicks EF, Barohn R, et al. Practice parameter: Immunotherapy for Guillain-Barré syndrome: report of the Quality Standards Subcommittee of the American Academy of Neurology. *Neurology*. 2003;61(6):736.
7. Elovaara I, Apostolski S, van Doorn P, et al. EFNS guidelines for the use of intravenous immunoglobulin in treatment of neurological diseases: EFNS task force on the use of intravenous immunoglobulin in treatment of neurological diseases. *Eur J Neurol*. 2008;15(9):893–908.
8. Criteria for diagnosis of Guillain-Barré syndrome. *Ann Neurol*. 1978;3(6):565.
9. Golestaneh L, Mokrzycki MH. Vascular access in therapeutic apheresis: update 2013. *J Clin Apher*. 2013;28(1):64–72.

IVIG versus Plasma Exchange for Myasthenia Gravis

KIMBERLY R. ROBESON

> ... IVIg has comparable efficacy to [plasma exchange] in the treatment of patients with moderate to severe [myasthenia gravis] ...
>
> —BARTH ET AL.[1]

Research Question: Both intravenous immunoglobulin (IVIG) and plasma exchange (PE) appear useful in treating patients with worsening myasthenia gravis (MG). However, which treatment is more effective?[1]

Funding: Talecris Biotherapeutics Inc.

Year Study Began: 2007

Year Study Published: 2011

Study Location: University Health Network, Toronto General Hospital, Toronto, Canada.

Who Was Studied: Patients aged ≥18 years with moderate to severe MG, defined as a Quantitative Myasthenia Gravis Score (QMGS) >10.5, and worsening weakness requiring a change in treatment modality as determined by a neuromuscular expert.

Who Was Excluded: Patients with MG worsening secondary to concurrent medications (e.g., aminoglycosides) or infection, other disorders causing weakness, poorly controlled hypertension, pregnancy, or who were breastfeeding were excluded. Patients were required to be on a stable dose of corticosteroids for the 2 weeks prior to screening. In addition, patients with known immunoglobulin A deficiency, active renal or hepatic disease, clinically significant cardiac disease, known hyperviscosity or hypercoaguable state, a history of anaphylaxis, severe systemic response to IVIG or albumin, or known refractory status to previous IVIG or PE were also excluded as these factors would have prohibited the use of one or both treatment options.

How Many Patients: 84

Study Overview: See Figure 23.1 for a summary of the study's design.

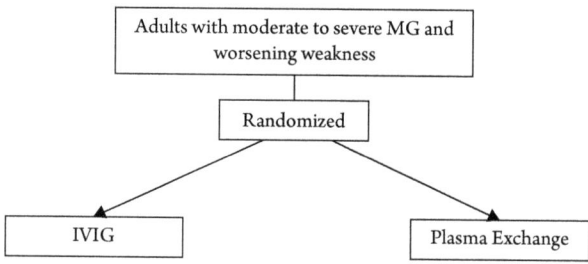

Figure 23.1 Summary of Study Design.

Study Intervention: Patients in the IVIG group received 1 g/kg/day of IVIG (Gamunex, Talecris Biotherapeutics, Mississauga, Canada) for 2 consecutive days. They were pretreated with Benadryl 50 mg PO and Tylenol 1,000 mg PO to reduce potential side effects of IVIG. Patients in the PE group received 1.0 plasma volume exchanges with 5% albumin replacement fluid. Five plasma exchange procedures were performed every second day with breaks allowed over the weekend.

Follow-Up: 60 days.

Endpoints: Primary outcome: change in the QMGS from baseline to day 14 after full treatment. Secondary outcomes: change in the QMGS from baseline to days 21 and 28; change in single-fiber electromyography (SFEMG) jitter; abnormal pairs; blocking pairs; percentage decrement in repetitive nerve stimulation (RNS) from baseline to days 14, 21, and 28; postintervention status at days 14, 21, and 28; and change in acetylcholine receptor antibody titers from baseline to days 28 and 60. Need for ICU admission, positive pressure ventilation or intubation, any hospitalization, and additional therapy for MG were also assessed.

The QMGS is a 13-item scale that grades degree of weakness from 0 (none) to 3 (severe). Bulbar symptoms, pulmonary function, and extremity strength are all assessed.[2]

RESULTS

- The change in QMGS at day 14 from baseline was 4.0, without significant difference between treatment groups (see Table 23.1).
- Dropout rate was the same for both treatment arms and both treatments were well tolerated.
- The presence of AChR antibodies and greater baseline disease severity predicted a better response to therapy (with either modality).

Table 23.1. SUMMARY OF THE TRIAL'S KEY FINDINGS

Outcome	Group		P Value
	IVIG	PLEX	
Change in QMGS at day 14	3.2 ±4.1	4.7 ±4.9	0.13
% responders (change > 3.5 on QMGS)	51%	57%	0.5
Postintervention status (% improved)	69%	65%	0.74

Criticisms and Limitations: This was a single-center study and included no patients who were in respiratory distress or intubated. The dropout rate in the study was relatively high in both arms. The primary outcome was not one that measured the functional abilities or status of the patient.

IVIG and PE were both readily available for patients in this study and most patients received PE through peripheral venous access.[3] However, in "real world" settings there may be a delay in starting PLEX, which may require central vascular access and availability of specialized equipment.

Patients were evaluated at 14, 21 and 28 days after completion of treatment. PE requires 5 exchanges, often performed over the course of 2 weeks. In this study, a complete round of IVIG was administered in 2 days. Therefore, patients in the PE group were evaluated later after initial exacerbation than patients in the IVIG group.

Other Relevant Studies and Information:

- Gajdos et al.[4] performed a randomized controlled trial to evaluate 3 days of PE versus 2 doses of IVIG for treatment of acute myasthenic worsening. This study showed no difference among the three treatments but a full course of PE was not administered.
- Stricker et al.[5] reported that PE was superior to IVIG in a small, uncontrolled series of patients with an acute exacerbation of MG.
- Ronager et al[6] studied 12 patients with MG in a controlled crossover study of PLEX and IVIG and observed no difference in outcomes at 1 month, although PLEX worked more rapidly.

Summary and Implications: Immunomodulation for MG can be accomplished with either IVIG or PE. Therefore, availability of treatment options and patient's comorbidities should all be considered when choosing a therapy for worsening myasthenia gravis.

CLINICAL CASE: IVIG VERSUS PE IN PATIENTS WITH MYASTHENIA GRAVIS

Case History:
A 60-year-old woman with a history of acetylcholine receptor autoantibody positive myasthenia gravis is evaluated in clinic. She has had difficulty managing her disease and has been unable to taper prednisone below 40 mg per day without worsening symptoms. She reports worsening ptosis and diplopia, as well as new shortness of breath and dysphagia since her last visit 1 month ago.

On examination, her negative inspiratory force (NIF) is 28 cm H_2O, and her vital capacity is 1.2 liters. She has fatigable ptosis and reports diplopia at baseline and on end-gaze in all directions. Her voice is dysphonic and she has bifacial weakness, resulting in a "myasthenic snarl." Neck flexion, deltoid, and iliopsoas strength are initially 5/5 (MRC scale), but fatigue to 4/5 with repetitive testing.

Based on the results of this trial, how should you treat this patient?

Suggested Answer:
This trial establishes that IVIG and PE have comparable efficacy in the treatment of worsening MG. Availability of treatment options, the patient's comorbidity profile, and side effects of treatments should all be considered when choosing one therapy over another. This patient's worsening bulbar symptoms and declining NIF are concerning for impending neuromuscular respiratory failure. Therefore, in the absence of comorbidities that would preclude one of the options, she should receive whichever treatment can be administered more quickly.

References

1. Barth D, Nabavi Nouri M, Ng E, Nwe P, Bril V. Comparison of IVIg and PLEX in patients with myasthenia gravis. *Neurology.* 2011;76:2017–2023.
2. Tindall RS, Rollins JA, Phillips JT, Greenlee RG, Wells L, Belendiuk G. Preliminary results of a double-blind, randomized, placebo-controlled trial of cyclosporine in myasthenia gravis. *N Engl J Med.* 1987;316:719–724.
3. Ebadi H, Barth D, Bril V. Safety of plasma exchange therapy in patients with myasthenia gravis. *Muscle Nerve.* 2013;47(4):510–514.
4. Gajdos P Chevret S, Clair B, Tranchant C, Chastang C. Clinical trial of plasma exchange and high-dose intravenous immunoglobulin in myasthenia gravis: Myasthenia Gravis Clinical Study Group. *Ann Neurol.* 1997;41:789–796.
5. Stricker RB, Kwiatkowska BJ, Habis JA, Kiprov DD. Myasthenic crisis: Response to plasmapheresis following failure of intravenous gamma-globulin. *Arch. Neurol.* 1993;50:837–840.
6. Rønager J, Ravnborg M, Hermansen I, Vorstrup S. Immunoglobulin treatment versus plasma exchange in patients with chronic moderate to severe myasthenia gravis. *Artif Organs.* 2001;25:967–973.

24
Riluzole for Amyotrophic Lateral Sclerosis

BRIAN MAC GRORY

> Whatever its mechanism of action, riluzole may be able to modify the course of amyotrophic lateral sclerosis.
> —The ALS/Riluzole Study Group[1]

Research Question: Is there a benefit in terms of survival and functional status to treating patients with amyotrophic lateral sclerosis (ALS) with riluzole, a modulator of glutamatergic transmission?[1]

Funding: Rhône-Poulenc Rorer, pharmaceutical company, now part of Aventis.

Year Study Began: 1990

Year Study Published: 1994

Study Location: 7 centers in France.

Who Was Studied: Outpatients 20–75 years old with probable or definite ALS.[2]

Who Was Excluded: Patients more than 5 years since the onset of symptoms, those with a forced vital capacity <60 liters, those with a tracheostomy, a concomitant life-threatening diagnoses, or pregnancy. Also excluded were those with signs of conduction blocks of motor nerves, sensory nerves, or both on electromyography; paraproteinemia on immunoelectrophoresis; "substantial lesions accounting for the clinical signs on imaging studies";[1] or signs of dementia.

How Many Patients: 155

Study Overview: See Figure 24.1 for a summary of the study's design.

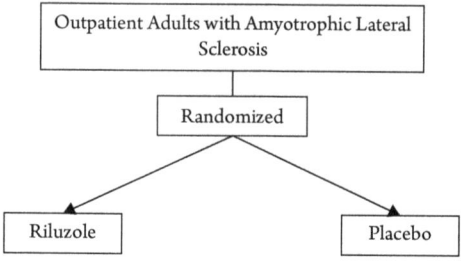

Figure 24.1 Summary of the Study's Design.

Study Intervention: Patients enrolled in the trial were either treated with riluzole 50 mg twice daily orally or identical-appearing placebo tablets (also given twice daily).

Follow-Up: 12 months. Of note, patients continued on study medication after 12 months, until the analysis of efficacy was performed in March 1992.

Endpoints: Primary endpoints were (1) survival and (2) changes in functional status at 12 months. The survival rate was determined as a composite of death and tracheostomy insertion. Functional status was quantified with a previously validated rating scale composed of limb function, bulbar function, results of clinical examination, and reported symptoms. This was measured every 2 months. Secondary endpoints were (1) a muscle testing score, respiratory indices, clinical global impression of change scale, and subjective evaluations of symptoms. Respiratory function was formally assessed every 6 months. Liver function tests and muscle enzymes were monitored regularly as well.

RESULTS

- Overall, 155 patients were included, of whom 32 had bulbar-onset disease and 123 had limb-onset disease.
- After 12 months of treatment, 74% of the riluzole group were alive, as opposed to 58% of the placebo group ($P = 0.014$).
- Riluzole reduced mortality by 38.6% at 12 months and 19.4% at 21 months (the end of the entire placebo-controlled period).

- Among patients with bulbar-onset disease, 73% of patients in the riluzole group were alive at 12 months, versus 35% of the placebo group ($P = 0.014$).
- Among patients with limb-onset disease, 74% of patients in the riluzole group were still alive at 12 months, as opposed to 64% of patients in the placebo group. This trend was not statistically significant ($P = 0.17$).
- Among all functional scores (e.g., limb function, bulbar function, muscle strength) measured in the trial, only the rate of deterioration of muscle strength was slower in the riluzole group than in the placebo group ($P = 0.028$).
- Twenty-seven patients in the riluzole group discontinued treatment versus 17 in the placebo group. Of the patients who withdrew because of perceived adverse drug events, a greater fraction were located in the riluzole group (19/27) versus the placebo group (9/15).

Criticisms and Limitations: When 24 patients who turned out subsequently not to meet criteria for enrollment were removed from the analysis, the study lacked sufficient power to demonstrate a survival advantage. These patients were evenly distributed between the two groups (11 were in the riluzole group and 13 were in the placebo group). The trial succeeded in showing a significant survival benefit only in those patients who had bulbar-onset disease. The mechanism of riluzole in ALS remains poorly understood.

Other Relevant Studies and Information:

- A subsequent double-blind, placebo-controlled study of 959 patients with ALS for less than 5 years examined the difference between placebo, 50 mg riluzole per day, 100 mg of riluzole per day, and 200 mg riluzole per day.[3] This trial confirmed a survival advantage with riluzole and suggested the optimal dose is 100 mg per day.
- A trial from Japan published in 1997 failed to demonstrate a benefit to riluzole over placebo in terms of disease progression but—unlike other trials—the authors did not report survival rates.[4]
- The American Academy of Neurology recommends riluzole as therapy for reducing progression of ALS.[5]

Summary and Implications: Riluzole increased rates of survival and decreased the rate of muscle strength deterioration in patients with ALS. This increased survival was most pronounced in those with bulbar-onset disease, and the trial failed to show a significant benefit for those with limb-onset disease. Based on the results of this and other studies, current guidelines recommend riluzole for the treatment of ALS.

CLINICAL CASE: RILUZOLE IN ALS

Case History:
A 58-year-old gentleman with no past medical history is referred to a neurologist for investigation of a 4-month history of progressive weakness in his legs—more pronounced in his right than left—as well as worsening dysarthria. A thorough physical examination suggests the presence of both upper and lower motor neuron signs in his extremities. Imaging of his brain and spine is within normal limits. Electromyography is performed, revealing evidence of both acute and chronic denervation diffusely as well as prominent fasciculation potentials, supportive of a diagnosis of ALS.

Based on the results of this study, how should this patient be treated?

Suggested Answer:
This trial suggested a benefit to treatment with 50 mg riluzole twice daily. This benefit manifested as increased interval to death or tracheostomy insertion that was most pronounced in those with bulbar-onset disease. This gentleman should be started on riluzole at a dose of 50 mg twice daily, with measurement of baseline liver function tests (LFTs). LFTs should be checked on a monthly basis for the first 3 months and every 3 months thereafter. He should also be counseled on the most common side effects of riluzole, which include gastrointestinal upset, dizziness, and asthenia.

References

1. Bensimon G, Lacomblez L, Meininger V. A controlled trial of riluzole in amyotrophic lateral sclerosis. ALS/Riluzole Study Group. *N Engl J Med.* 1994;330(9): 585–591.
2. Swash M, Leigh N. Criteria for diagnosis of familial amyotrophic lateral sclerosis. European FALS Collaborative Group. *Neuromuscul Disord.* 1992;2(1):7–9.
3. Lacomblez L, Bensimon G, Leigh PN, Guillet P, Meininger V. Dose-ranging study of riluzole in amyotrophic lateral sclerosis. Amyotrophic Lateral Sclerosis/Riluzole Study Group II. *Lancet.* 1996;347(9013):1425–1431.

4. Yanagisawa N, Tohgi H, Mizuno Y, Kowa H, Kimuma J, et al. Efficacy and safety of riluzole in patients with amyotrophic lateral sclerosis: double-blind placebo-controlled study in Japan. *Igakuno Ayumi.* 1997:851–66.
5. Miller RG, Jackson CE, Kasarskis EJ, et al. Practice parameter update: the care of the patient with amyotrophic lateral sclerosis: drug, nutritional, and respiratory therapies (an evidence-based review): report of the Quality Standards Subcommittee of the American Academy of Neurology. *Neurology.* 2009;73(15):1218–1226.

SECTION IX

Neuro-Oncology

25
Radiotherapy Plus Temozolomide for Glioblastoma

AMY CHAN

> ... Addition of temozolomide to radiotherapy for newly diagnosed glioblastoma resulted in a clinically meaningful and statistically significant survival benefit with minimal additional toxicity.
> —STUPP ET AL.[1]

Research Question: The standard of care for newly diagnosed glioblastoma is surgical resection followed by adjuvant radiotherapy. What is the efficacy and safety of adjuvant temozolomide, given postoperatively in addition to radiotherapy?[1]

Funding: National Cancer Institute and Schering-Plough (Pharmaceutical) Corporation, Kenilworth, NJ.

Year Study Began: 2000

Year Study Published: 2005

Study Location: 85 institutions in 15 countries in Europe, Canada, and Australia.

Who Was Studied: Patients aged 18–70 years with newly diagnosed and histologically confirmed glioblastoma (WHO grade IV astrocytoma).

Who Was Excluded: Patients with a WHO performance status[2] ≥3; who required an increasing dose of corticosteroids; or who had inadequate hematological, renal, and hepatic function (absolute neutrophil count < 1,500/mm³; platelet count < 100,000/mm³; serum creatinine level or total serum bilirubin level > 1.5 times the upper limit of normal; or liver function values > 3 times the upper limit of normal).

How Many Patients: 573

Study Overview: See Figure 25.1 for a summary of the study design.

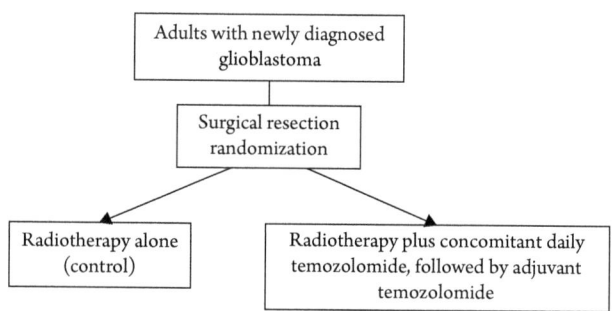

Figure 25.1 Summary of the Study's Design.

Study Intervention:

1. Radiotherapy consisted of fractional focal irradiation at a dose of 2 Gy per fraction delivered to the gross tumor volume with a 2–3 cm clinical margin given Monday to Friday, over 6 weeks for a total dose of 60 Gy.
2. Concomitant temozolomide was delivered at 75 mg/m²/day given 7 days per week from the first day of radiotherapy until the last day of radiotherapy, but for no longer than 49 days. This was given with

Pneumocystis carinii pneumonia prophylaxis (either with inhaled pentamidine or oral trimethoprim-sulfamethoxazole).
3. Adjuvant temozolomide was delivered after a 4-week break according to the standard 5-day schedule every 28 days. The dose was 150 mg/m^2 for the first cycle and then increased to 200 mg/m^2 beginning with the second cycle, up to 6 cycles, as long as there were no hematological toxic effects.

Follow-Up: Daily during radiotherapy and every 3 months thereafter with a median follow-up of 28 months.

Endpoints: Primary: overall survival. Secondary: (1) progression-free survival, according to the modified WHO criteria of <25% increase in tumor size, no new lesions, and no increased need for corticosteroid treatment; (2) safety, as graded according to the National Cancer Institute Common Toxicity Criteria, Version 2.0; (3) quality of life, as measured by a comprehensive evaluation including WHO performance status, Mini-Mental State Examination, and a quality-of-life questionnaire.

RESULTS

- At median follow-up of 28 months, 480 patients (84%) had died.
- The median survival benefit of patients in the radiotherapy-plus-temozolomide group was 2.5 months, with a 2-year survival rate of 26.5% versus 10.4% for the radiation-alone group (see Tables 25.1 & 25.2).
- The most common adverse event was moderate-to-severe fatigue.

Table 25.1. WORLD HEALTH ORGANIZATION PERFORMANCE STATUS

Score	Description
0	Fully active and more or less as you were before your illness
1	Cannot carry out heavy physical work, but can do anything else
2	Up and about more than half the day and can look after yourself, but are not well enough to work
3	In bed or sitting in a chair for more than half the day and you need some help in looking after yourself
4	In bed or a chair all the time and need a lot of looking after

Adapted from WHO Handbook for reporting cancer treatment, http://whqlibdoc.who.int/publications/9241700483.pdf.

Table 25.2. SUMMARY OF KEY FINDINGS

Outcome	Radiotherapy plus Temozolomide (n = 287)	Radiotherapy (n = 286)	P Value
Median overall survival (months)	14.6	12.1	<0.001
Overall survival			
At 18 months	39.4%	20.9%	
At 24 months	26.5%	10.4%	
Median progression-free survival (months)	6.9	5.0	<0.001
Progression-free survival			
At 18 months	18.4%	3.9%	
At 24 months	10.7%	1.5%	
Grade 3–4 hematologic toxicity			
Concomitant phase	7%	None	
Adjuvant phase	14%		
Severe infection	3%	2%	
Thromboembolic events	4%	5%	
Moderate-to-severe fatigue	33%	26%	

Criticisms and Limitations: Quality of life metrics were not reported. Whether the addition of chemotherapy increases the risk of radiotherapy-induced cognitive deficits cannot be assessed. Overall short survival also limits evaluation of late toxic effects, such as myelodysplastic syndrome or secondary leukemia. All of these metrics would be more relevant if treatment was to be used in patients with intermediate- or low-grade glioma, who have longer expected survival.

Other Relevant Studies and Information:

- A companion translational study, "*MGMT* Gene Silencing and Benefit from Temozolomide in Glioblastoma,"[3] further characterized the molecular profile of patients (with methylated *MGMT* promoter) who derived most of the benefits. This finding could help tailor therapy to patients most likely to benefit from temozolomide.
- Other aberrant activation or suppression of cellular signals leading to resistance to radiation and chemotherapy currently being investigated include antiangiogenic agents (bevacizumab, enzastaurin), inhibitors of the epidermal growth-factor receptor tyrosine kinase (gefitinib and

erlotinib), mammalian target of rapamycin (temsirolimus, everolimus) and integrin (cilengitide)[4]
- During guideline development for management of newly diagnosed glioblastoma, the Joint Section for Tumors of the AANS and CNS classified this prospective, randomized trial with clearly defined histopathology and adequate power as class I evidence. This had translated into a level I recommendation as summarized below.[5]

Summary and Implications: The addition of temozolomide to radiotherapy early in the course of glioblastoma provides a significant, albeit modest (2.5 months) survival benefit. Continuous administration of an alkylating agent like temozolomide is thought to provide synergy by depleting the *MGMT* protein that may otherwise be induced for DNA-repair by radiotherapy. The 2009 guidelines[5] currently recommend concurrent and postirradiation temozolomide as an adjuvant to surgery in patients with newly diagnosed glioblastoma and adequate systemic health, aged 18–70 years.

CLINICAL CASE: CONCOMITANT AND ADJUVANT CHEMOTHERAPY FOR GLIOBLASTOMA

Case History:
A 68-year-old man was brought to the hospital after suffering the first seizure of his life while watching TV. When his wife asked him a question, he answered in "gibberish." He then had a generalized convulsion in the emergency room. Neuroimaging revealed a left hemispheric infiltrative mass.

An MRI of the brain with contrast and functional MRI obtained as preoperation planning showed an ill-defined T2/FLAIR hyperintense mass centered in the lateral aspect of the left temporal lobe. There was surrounding mass effect, contrast enhancement, and restricted diffusion.

The patient underwent surgical resection of the mass. Histopathology was diagnostic of a WHO grade IV astrocytoma (glioblastoma). Based on the results of the above trial, would you treat this patient with radiation and concurrent temozolomide?

Suggested Answer:
Yes. This patient has a histologically proven glioblastoma and a good performance status (WHO 0). The trial showed a statistically significant and clinical meaningful survival benefit with concurrent temozolomide with minimal additional toxicity.

The most common side effect to be expected would be fatigue. Hematological toxicity should be monitored. Patient receiving temozolomide should receive *Pneumocystis carinii* pneumonia prophylaxis, as in the trial.

References

1. Stupp R, Mason WP, van den Bent MJ, et al. Radiotherapy plus concomitant and adjuvant temozolomide for glioblastoma. *NEJM*. 2005;352(10):987–996.
2. WHO Handbook for reporting cancer treatment. http://whqlibdoc.who.int/publications/9241700483.pdf
3. Hegi M, Diserens AC, Gorlia T, et al. MGMT gene silencing and benefit from temozolomide in glioblastoma. *New Engl. J. Med.* 2005;352(10):997–1003.
4. Minniti G, Muni, Lanzetta G, Marchetti P, Enrici RM. Chemotherapy for glioblastoma: current treatment and future perspectives for cytotoxic and targeted agents. *Anticancer Res.* 29(12):5171–5184.
5. Olson JJ, Fadul CE, Brat DJ, Mukundan S, Ryken TC. Management of newly diagnosed glioblastoma: guidelines development, value and application. *J Neurooncol.* 2009;93(1):1–23.

26

Methylated *MGMT* Gene Promoter and Response to Temozolomide for Glioblastoma

JOSHUA LOVINGER

> MGMT promoter methylation is associated with a favorable outcome after temozolomide chemotherapy in patients with newly diagnosed glioblastoma.
>
> —Hegi et al.[1]

Research Question: Does epigenetic silencing of the O^6-methylguanine-DNA methyltransferase (*MGMT*) DNA-repair gene by promoter methylation confer benefit to temozolomide (TMZ; an alkylating chemotherapy) in patients with glioblastoma?[1]

Funding: European Organisation for Research and Treatment of Cancer (EORTC) and National Cancer Institute of Canada (NCIC). Schering-Plough, a pharmaceutical company, provided the study drug.

Year Study Began: 2000

Year Study Published: 2005

Study Location: Patients from 66 of the 85 centers (in 15 countries) that participated in the larger parent trial of temozolomide and radiotherapy versus radiotherapy alone for glioblastoma.[2]

Who Was Studied: Patients aged 18–70 years with newly diagnosed and histologically confirmed glioblastoma (WHO grade IV astrocytoma).

Who Was Excluded: Patients with poor WHO performance status[3] (>2) or predefined inadequate hematologic, renal, or hepatic function. The WHO performance status is also known as the Eastern Cooperative Oncology Group (ECOG) performance status. It is a functional score, graded 0–5, with 0 = asymptomatic (fully active) and 5 = dead. In general, the higher the WHO/ECOG performance status grade, the worse the outcome, either with or without treatment; as a result, oncology trials frequently limit inclusion to patients with scores of 0–2. Patients who were receiving corticosteroids had to receive a stable or decreasing dose for at least 14 days before randomization. In addition, the study included only those patients (of the parent study population of 573) for whom adequate tumor tissue was available.

How Many Patients: 206

Study Overview: See Figure 26.1 for a summary of the study's design.

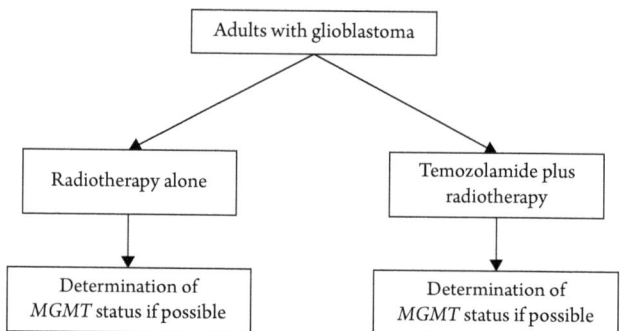

Figure 26.1 Summary of the Study's Design.

Study Intervention: Patients in the radiotherapy-alone group (control) received a dose of 2 Gy per fraction given once daily for 5 days per week over a period of 6 weeks, for a total dose of 60 Gy. Patients in the experimental group received the alkylating agent TMZ at a dose of 75 mg/m^2 of body surface area daily, given 7 days a week from the first day of standard fractionated radiotherapy (60 Gy) until the last day of radiotherapy, but for no longer than 49 days. After a 4-week break, patients were then to receive adjuvant TMZ at a dose of 150–200 mg/m^2 of body surface area for 5 days of every 28-day cycle after radiotherapy, for up to 6 cycles. In the case of tumor progression, second-line chemotherapy was administered at the investigator's discretion. MGMT status was determined using methylation-specific polymerase chain reaction testing on DNA from glioblastoma samples.

Follow-Up: 2 years.

Endpoints: Comparison of overall and progression-free Kaplan-Meier survival curves.

RESULTS

- Irrespective of treatment assignment, there was a difference in the 2-year survival between patients with a methylated *MGMT* promoter versus with an unmethylated promoter (55% risk reduction with a methylated *MGMT* promoter, $P < 0.001$). Median overall survival with methylated promoter was 18.2 months, versus 12.2 months among those with an unmethylated promoter.
- Patients with the methylated *MGMT* promoter who received TMZ plus radiotherapy had better outcomes than those receiving radiotherapy alone; the benefit of TMZ was less apparent among those without the methylated *MGMT* promoter (see Table 26.1).
- A confounding factor in the analysis of overall survival was administration of second-line chemotherapy after disease progression; in the radiotherapy alone group, 59.7% received TMZ as salvage chemotherapy.

Table 26.1. SUMMARY OF THE TRIAL'S KEY FINDINGS

Outcome[a]	Radiotherapy	TMZ + Radiotherapy	P Value[b]
Methylated *MGMT* promoter			
Progression-free survival	5.9	10.3	0.001
Overall survival	15.3	21.7	0.007
Unmethylated *MGMT* promoter			
Progression-free survival	4.4	5.3	0.02
Overall survival	11.8	12.7	0.06

[a] All outcome values are median duration (of survival) in months.
[b] For difference between survival curves.

Criticisms and Limitations: The patients were relatively healthy, all under 70 years old with a performance status of ≤2. Only 3.4% of patients in the analysis had a diagnostic biopsy alone (without debulking surgery). Perhaps elderly patients >70 years, those with a poor performance status, and those whose tumors could not be debulked would derive less benefit from the addition of TMZ, even in the setting of a methylated *MGMT* promoter.[4]

The technique of methylation-specific PCR proved to be a difficult one, highly dependent on tissue quality, and difficult to standardize for widespread use. Other methods of determining *MGMT* promoter methylation status, such as immunohistochemistry, were thought to be less reliable and were not addressed. Of the initial 307 patients for whom adequate tumor samples were available in the parent study, *MGMT* promoter methylation status could only be determined in 206.

As patients with tumors with methylated *MGMT* promoters had increased overall survival irrespective of treatment, there was also criticism that the predictive role of *MGMT* in determining response to alkylating chemotherapy was overstated.

Other Relevant Studies and Information:

- Elderly patients with glioblastoma are not typically given combined modality treatment with both chemotherapy and radiotherapy due to reduced tolerability of the combination, as well as an association with decreased benefit from chemotherapy and increasing risk of cognitive side effects from cranial irradiation. In 2012, two independent randomized trials looked at elderly glioma patients (a group excluded from Stupp et al. and Hegi et al.)[1,2]. The NOA-08 trial[5] (patients were >65 years and had anaplastic astrocytoma or glioblastoma) demonstrated that chemotherapy alone with TMZ in patients with a methylated *MGMT* promoter was noninferior to radiotherapy alone, with a predictive role for methylation status. The Nordic trial[6] (patients were >60 years and had glioblastoma only) compared the use of TMZ, hypofractionated radiotherapy, and standard radiotherapy in newly diagnosed glioblastoma. The study supported not only the overall prognostic role of *MGMT* promoter methylation, but also its role in predicting response to TMZ.

Summary and Implications: This study demonstrated *MGMT* promoter methylation as a favorable prognostic factor in patients with glioblastoma. It also suggested that methylation status may help to predict which patients are most likely to benefit from alkylating chemotherapy.

CLINICAL CASE: METHYLATED *MGMT* GENE PROMOTER AND RESPONSE TO TEMOZOLOMIDE IN GLIOBLASTOMA

Case History:

A 60-year-old right-handed man is brought to the emergency room after suffering a first-time seizure. His family accompanies him. They report that he had been complaining of headaches and nausea for the preceding 3 weeks, but no other symptoms.

An MRI with gadolinium demonstrates an irregular, heterogeneously enhancing mass with surrounding edema in his right frontal lobe.

He is brought to the operating room where debulking of the tumor is performed. The frozen section is consistent with glioblastoma. Methylation analysis of the *MGMT* promoter is positive.

How should this man be treated? What information regarding prognosis can you provide the patient and his family?

Suggested Answer:

Hegi et al. demonstrated that patients with newly diagnosed glioblastoma with a methylated *MGMT* promoter have increased progression-free and overall survival compared to those with an unmethylated promoter. The patient has a number of good prognostic features (e.g., the tumor could be debulked, has had minimal symptoms, and is likely to have a good performance status). Because of the methylated *MGMT* promoter, he is likely to benefit from the addition of an alkylating chemotherapy like TMZ to standard radiotherapy after surgery.

References

1. Hegi M, Diserens AC, Gorlia T, et al. MGMT gene silencing and benefit from temozolomide in glioblastoma. *New Engl. J. Med.* 2005;352(10):997–1003.
2. Stupp R, Mason WP, van den Bent MJ, et al. Radiotherapy plus concomitant and adjuvant temozolomide for glioblastoma. *NEJM.* 2005;352(10):987–996.
3. Oken MM, Creech RH, Tormey DC, et al. Toxicity and response criteria of the Eastern Cooperative Oncology Group. *Am J Clin Oncol.* 1982;5(6):649–655.
4. DeAngelis LM. Chemotherapy for brain tumors—a new beginning. *NEJM.* 2005;352(10):1036–1038.
5. Wick W, Platten M, Meisner C. et al. Temozolomide chemotherapy alone versus radiotherapy alone for malignant astrocytoma in the elderly; the NOA-08 randomised, phase 3 trial. *Lancet Oncol.* 2012;13(7):707–715.
6. Malmström A, Grønberg BH, Marosi C, et al. Temozolomide versus standard 6-week radiotherapy versus hypofractionated radiotherapy in patients older than 60 years with glioblastoma: the Nordic randomised, phase 3 trial. *Lancet Oncol.* 2012;13(9):916–926.

SECTION X

Neuro-Ophthalmology

27

Steroids for Acute Optic Neuritis
The Optic Neuritis Treatment Trial

MARY A. BAILEY

> Intravenous methylprednisolone followed by oral prednisone speeds the recovery of visual loss due to optic neuritis and results in slightly better vision at six months.
> —BECK ET AL.[1]

Research Question: Is there a benefit to treating acute optic neuritis with either oral corticosteroids alone or intravenously followed by oral corticosteroids?[1]

Funding: National Eye Institute, National Institute of Health.

Year Study Began: 1988

Year Study Published: 1992

Study Location: 15 clinics throughout the United States.

Who Was Studied: Patients between ages 18–46 that had clinical evidence of an acute, unilateral optic neuritis of ≤8 days in duration.

Who Was Excluded: "Patients with a previous optic neuritis in the affected eye or those who had a systemic disease, other than multiple sclerosis [MS], that may cause optic neuritis."[1]

How Many Patients: 457

Study Overview: See Figure 27.1 for a summary of the study's design.

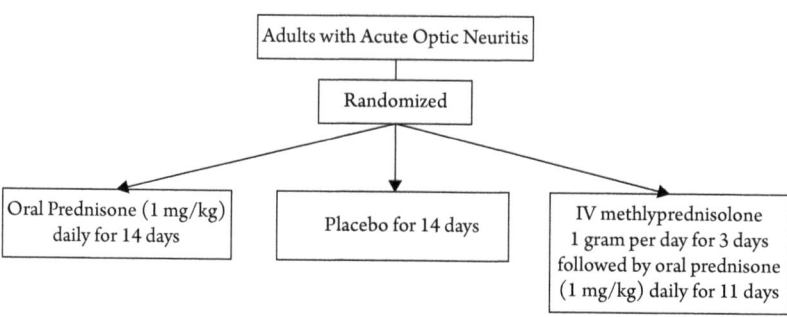

Figure 27.1 Summary of ONTT's Design.

Study Intervention: Patients were randomized into three treatment groups. The first group was treated with 14 days of oral placebo. The second group was treated with 14 days of oral prednisone (1mg/kg of body weight) daily for 14 days. The third group was treated with "1 gram daily of IV methylprednisolone for 3 days followed by oral prednisone (1mg/kg of body weight) daily for 11 days."[1]

Follow-Up: 6 months.

Endpoints: Primary outcome: visual field and "contrast sensitivity" ("the eye's ability to recognize targets with low contrast"). Secondary outcomes: visual acuity ("the eye's ability to resolve high-contrast small targets") and color vision.[1]

RESULTS

- "Visual function recovered faster in the IV methylprednisolone group as compared to the placebo group" (see Table 27.1).
- "At 6 months, the IV methylprednisolone group had better visual fields, contrast sensitivity, and color vision."
- There was no difference in outcome between the placebo group and the oral prednisone group.

- The rate of a new optic neuritis event in either eye was greater in the oral prednisone group versus the placebo group. This was not the case in the IV methylprednisolone group.

Table 27.1. SUMMARY OF "RESULTS COMPARING RECOVERY RATES IN THE STEROID GROUPS WITH RATES IN THE PLACEBO GROUP"[a]

	Visual Acuity	Contrast Sensitivity	Visual Field
Methylprednisolone (adjusted)	2.93 ($P = 0.09$)	5.91 ($P = 0.02$)	16.27 ($P = 0.0001$)
Prednisone (adjusted)	0.06 ($P = 0.39$)	0.75 ($P = 0.39$)	3.16 ($P = 0.08$)

[a] The numbers in this chart represent the chi-square statistic as calculated by the Kruskal-Wallis Test, with larger values simply reflecting a smaller probability that the difference between the recovery rates for the listed treatment arm versus placebo is due to pure chance. Corresponding P values are listed in parentheses as well.

Criticisms and Limitations: The patients in the IV methylprednisolone group were not blinded; however, the other two groups were. There was a delay in treatment from symptom onset of up to 8 days in some patients, resulting in variable lag until treatment initiation. There was no group tested with only IV methylprednisolone (without additional oral prednisone), which is a treatment method widely used in clinical practice to treat acute optic neuritis.

Other Relevant Studies and Information:

- Multiple follow-up studies have been done since the original publication of the Optic Neuritis Treatment Trial (ONTT). The 15-year follow-up study showed that long-term outcomes for acute optic neuritis were favorable, with 72% of initially affected eyes having a visual acuity ≥20/20.[2]
- Another follow-up study to the ONTT looked at the characteristics of the original study participants to determine "the clinical profile of acute optic neuritis." This study demonstrated that in most cases of acute optic neuritis the visual loss was accompanied by pain, and in only about one-third of the patients was there swelling of the optic disc.[3]
- The ONTT has been influential in how MS exacerbations are treated. Despite most other studies of MS and IV steroids not showing a benefit over oral steroid treatment (see Chapter 11), it is common practice to treat acute MS flares with IV corticosteroids.

Summary and Implications: This study concluded that treatment with IV methylprednisolone followed by oral prednisone for acute optic neuritis had better outcomes at 6 months than placebo and oral prednisone–only groups. It also found that treating with oral prednisone alone potentially "increases the risk of a new episodes of optic neuritis."[1] These findings support the use of IV corticosteroids and should dissuade physicians from treating with oral steroids alone.

CLINICAL CASE: STEROIDS FOR ACUTE OPTIC NEURITIS

Case History:
A 27-year-old woman developed pain with movement with accompanying darkening and blurring of the vision in her right eye. On exam she was found to have an afferent pupillary defect and a visual acuity of 20/100. Her baseline vision is 20/20 in both eyes without correction. She had no prior episodes of optic neuritis and no other medical conditions. On fundoscopic exam she was found to have optic disc pallor and papilledema. CT of her head was negative for any acute intracranial process. The treating physician diagnosed her with acute optic neuritis and planned to admit her to the hospital for 3 days of IV methylprednisolone treatment, as well as a workup for possible MS. However, the patient was scheduled to leave the next day on a business trip and asked if there was any oral medication she could take that would prevent her from having to change her plans.

How would you treat her acute optic neuritis, and how would you explain the benefits of intravenous versus oral steroids?

Suggested Answer:
The patient is suffering from an acute optic neuritis as characterized by pain with eye movement, worsening of visual acuity, and an afferent pupillary defect. The ONTT demonstrated that treatment of acute optic neuritis with 3 days of IV methylprednisolone, followed by oral prednisone, resulted in better recovery of vision at 6 months as compared to patients treated with oral prednisone alone or placebo.

The physician should explain this data to the patient and emphasize that postponing her trip so that she can receive the IV methylprednisolone will likely have more of a long-term benefit.

References

1. Beck RW, Cleary PA, Anderson MM, et al. A randomized, controlled trial of corticosteroids in the treatment of acute optic neuritis. *NEJM*. 1992;326:581–588.
2. The Optic Neuritis Study Group. Visual function 15 years after optic neuritis: a final follow-up report from the Optic Neuritis Treatment Trial. *Ophthalmology*. 2008;115(6):1079–1082
3. The Optic Neuritis Study Group. The clinical profile of optic neuritis. Experience of the Optic Neuritis Treatment Trial. *Arch Ophthalmol*. 1991;109(12):1673–1678.

#　SECTION XI

Neuro-Otology

The Epley Maneuver for Benign Paroxysmal Positional Vertigo

BENJAMIN N. BLOND

> The Canalith Repositioning Procedure is designed to treat benign paroxysmal positional vertigo through induced out-migration of free-moving pathological densities in the endolymph of a semicircular canal, using timed head maneuvers and applied vibration ... CRP should be the initial procedure of choice for treatment of BPPV. It is cost-effective and provides timely resolution in a high percentage of cases.
>
> —EPLEY[1]

Research Question: Is the canalith repositioning procedure (CRP) effective for the treatment of benign paroxysmal positional vertigo (BPPV)?[1]

Funding: None listed.

Year Study Began: 1988

Year Study Published: 1992

Study Location: Portland Otologic Clinic, Portland, Oregon.

Who Was Studied: All adult patients with classic findings of BPPV and treated with CRP at the Portland Otologic clinic during the 30-month study period.

Who Was Excluded: 2 patients are reported as excluded because their initial CRP was started before the beginning of the research period. No other exclusion criteria were listed

How Many Patients: 30

Study Overview: See Figure 28.1 for a summary of the study design.

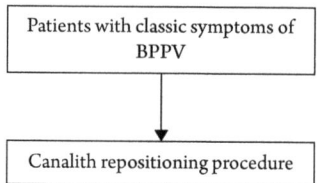

Figure 28.1 Summary of Study Design.

Study Intervention: Patients were premedicated with either a transdermal scopolamine patch the prior evening or 5 mg diazepam 1 hour prior to procedure. Patients underwent the 5-position cycle of repositioning (Figure 28.2). This was repeated until nystagmus was absent or until no progress was apparent during the last 2 trials. The timing of position changes was determined by the rate of change of observed nystagmus and was typically 6–13 seconds in each position. If nystagmus was not observed after a given position change, the timing was based on the last observed nystagmus for the remainder of the positioning cycle. Patients also had vibration applied to the ipsilateral mastoid area with a 700 Hz electromagnetic bone conduction vibrator for at least one positioning cycle and then with a handheld 80 Hz vibrator for at least 1 cycle. Patients were advised to keep their heads relatively upright for 48 hours following the procedure. CRP was repeated as necessary at weekly intervals until vertigo resolved and the Dix-Hallpike maneuver was negative.

Follow-Up: 10 months.

Endpoints: Response to treatment was characterized by a 4-point scale as detailed in Table 28.1. Recurrences and the success of repeat treatments were also recorded.

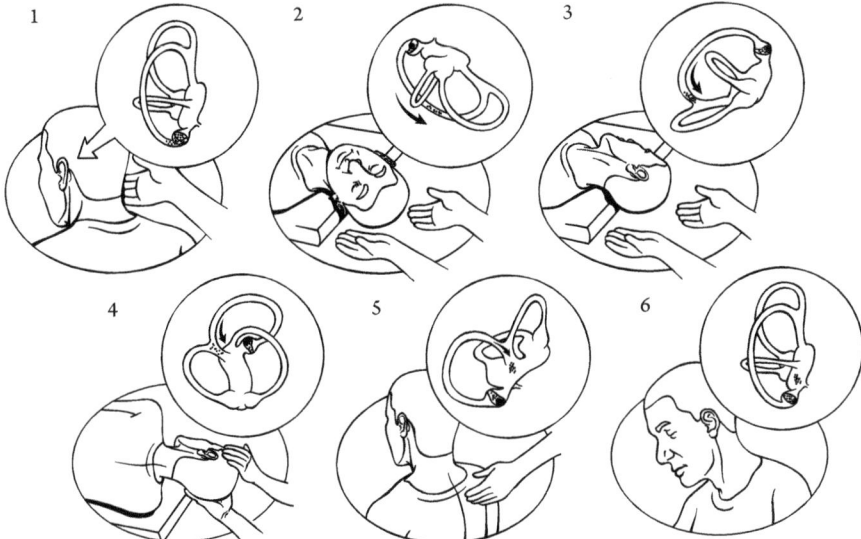

Figure 28.2 This diagram demonstrates the canalith repositioning procedure as it would be performed for left BPPV, as described and diagramed by Epley (1992). The examiner is instructed to pause at each position until nystagmus has nearly resolved. The steps may be repeated in order until there is no nystagmus at any position: (1) first the patient is seated on the exam table; (2) the head is placed over the end of the table, 45° to the left, so that the canaliths gravitate to the center of the posterior semicircular canal; (3) the head remains tilted downward as it is rotated 45° degrees to the right, so that the canaliths reach the common crus; (4) the head and body are then rotated until facing downward 135° from the supine position, allowing the canaliths to traverse the common crus; (5) while keeping the head turned to the right, the patient is then brought back to a sitting position, causing the canaliths to enter the utricle; (6) the head is then turned forward, with the chin turned down 20°. (Illustration by Michael T. Loscalzo)

Table 28.1. RESPONSE TO CANALITH REPOSITIONING PROCEDURE

I	All vertigo (and nystagmus) resolved
II	BPPV resolved, other vertigo remains: Free of positional vertigo and induced rotatory nystagmus, but nonpositional vertigo still present
III	Partially resolved: Positional vertigo symptoms significantly improved, though still present
IV	Same or worse: (none in this study)

Epley JM. The canalith repositioning procedure: for treatment of benign paroxysmal positional vertigo. *Otolaryngol Head Neck Surg.* 1992;107(3):399–404.

RESULTS

- Twenty-seven of 30 (90%) patients had complete resolution of vertigo (result category I) after initial treatment (see Table 28.2).
- Three of 30 (10%) patients had resolution of BPPV, but nonpositional vertigo remained (result category II) after initial treatment.
- BPPV recurred at least once in 9 patients (30%).
- Of 14 additional CRP treatments for recurrence, only 1 did not have a category I or II response.
- Overall, 43 of 44 courses of treatment with CRP resulted in resolution of BPPV.

Table 28.2. SUMMARY OF KEY FINDINGS

Result Category	Initial Treatment Result (30 Total)	Treatment of Recurrence Results (14 Total)	All Treatment Results (44 Total)
I All vertigo resolved	27 (90%)	12 (85.7%)	39 (88.6%)
II BPPV resolved/ other vertigo remains	3 (10%)	1 (7.1%)	4 (9.1%)
III Partially resolved	0	1 (7.1%)	1 (2.3%)
IV Same or worse	0	0	0

Epley JM. The canalith repositioning procedure: for treatment of benign paroxysmal positional vertigo. *Otolaryngol Head Neck Surg.* 1992;107(3):399–404.

Criticisms and Limitations: This initial study was limited by its nature as an single-center, uncontrolled case series, particularly since BPPV resolves spontaneously in many cases (15%–84% in some studies[2,3]). However, this study was the first evaluation of a promising technique for the treatment of BPPV, which has been validated by further research, as described below.

Other Relevant Studies and Information:

- Multiple subsequent studies have confirmed the efficacy of CRP in the treatment of posterior canal BPPV, including 5 randomized controlled trials, 4 with sham controls, where outcome was assessed

- by resolution of symptomatic vertigo and conversion to a negative response on Dix-Hallpike maneuver.[3-8]
- The Semont maneuver is an alternate repositioning technique, also used to treat posterior canal BPPV, but this technique has not been as well studied as CRP.[2,9]
- About 10%–17% of BPPV cases are caused by canalithiasis in the lateral semicircular canals, in which case the Epley maneuver is not effective. This condition is best diagnosed with the supine roll test and treated with the Lempert roll, forced prolonged positioning, and the Gufoni maneuver, although these therapies are less well established than CRP.[2,9]
- The use of medications prior to performing CRP typically has not been continued in subsequent studies or in general practice.[2,10]
- The use of mastoid region oscillation as described in the original manuscript has not been extensively investigated; however, available evidence suggests this intervention does not offer an additional benefit for BPPV.[10]
- The imposition of postural restrictions following the Epley maneuver is a more controversial subject. Most studies have demonstrated no statistically significant difference in outcomes with the use of postural restrictions. However, a recent Cochrane review found that pooling the data from these trials resulted in a statistically significant benefit in the use of postural restrictions as evidenced by conversion to a negative response on Dix-Hallpike maneuver, but the benefit is small, with a number needed to treat of 10.[10]

Summary and Implications: This study was the first to suggest a benefit of CRP, also known as the Epley maneuver, for treating BPPV. The technique is believed to work by guiding free canaliths out of the posterior semicircular canal, and the success of CRP provided significant support for the theory of canalithiasis, also championed by Dr. Epley, as a mechanism of BPPV. Epley's success in his case series inspired further research, including several randomized controlled trials, which demonstrated that CRP is effective at treating BPPV. CRP is now considered the first line of treatment for posterior canal BPPV.

CLINICAL CASE: TREATMENT OF BPPV

Case History:
A 50-year-old lady presents to your office with complaints of episodes of dizziness and nausea, described as room spinning, which last for less than one minute and occur with lying down in bed, extending the neck while reaching for objects on a shelf, or any other rapid change in head position.

As part of a complete neurologic exam, you perform a Dix-Hallpike maneuver and note rotatory nystagmus with the fast phase toward the right ear, which occurs after a latency of a few seconds, when the right ear is turned down. The nystagmus adapts with repeated testing.

Based on this, you are able to make a diagnosis of BPPV. What treatment may be offered to this patient?

Suggested Answer:
This patient has symptoms consistent with a diagnosis of BPPV, which is most commonly caused by posterior semicircular canal dysfunction. This study was the first to suggest a benefit of the Epley maneuver, also known as CRP, now considered the first line of treatment for BPPV. This noninvasive positioning technique has few adverse effects and has demonstrated effectiveness in treating BPPV, based on both subjective resolution of symptoms and objective resolution of abnormalities on performance of the Dix-Hallpike maneuver. CRP may need to be repeated to achieve resolution of symptoms. The benefit of imposing postural restrictions, such as requesting the patient to sleep upright for 24–48 hours and avoid lying on the affected ear for up to 5 days, is currently not clearly established, but may provide a small additional advantage.

References

1. Epley JM. The canalith repositioning procedure: for treatment of benign paroxysmal positional vertigo. *Otolaryngol Head Neck Surg.* 1992;107(3):399–404.
2. Fife TD. Positional dizziness. *Continuum (Minneap Minn).* 2012;18(5 Neuro-otology):1060–1085.
3. Froehling DA, Bowen JM, Mohr DN, et al. The canalith repositioning procedure for the treatment of benign paroxysmal positional vertigo: a randomized controlled trial. *Mayo Clin Proc.* 2000;75(7):695–700.
4. Hilton M, Pinder D. The Epley (canalith repositioning) manoeuvre for benign paroxysmal positional vertigo. *Cochrane Database Syst Rev.* 2004;(2):CD003162.
5. Lynn S, Pool A, Rose D, Brey R, Suman V. Randomized trial of the canalith repositioning procedure. *Otolaryngol Head Neck Surg.* 1995;113(6):712–720.

6. Munoz J, Miklea J, Howard M, Springate R, Kaczorowski J. Canalith repositioning maneuver for benign paroxysmal positional vertigo. *Can Fam Physician.* 2007;53:1048–1053.
7. von Brevern M, Seelig T, Radtke A, Tiel-Wilck K, Neuhauser H, Lempert T. Short-term efficacy of Epley's manoeuvre: a double-blind randomised trial. *J Neurol Neurosurg Psychiatry.* 2006;77:980–982.
8. Yimtae K, Srirompotong S, Srirompotong S, Sae-seaw P. A randomized trial of the canalith repositioning procedure. *Laryngoscope.* 2003;113:828–832.
9. Nguyen-Huynh AT. Evidence-based practice: management of vertigo. *Otolaryngol Clin North Am.* 2012;45(5):925–940.
10. Hunt WT, Zimmermann EF, Hilton MP. Modifications of the Epley (canalith repositioning) manoeuvre for posterior canal benign paroxysmal positional vertigo (BPPV). *Cochrane Database Syst Rev.* 2012;4:CD008675.

SECTION XII

Sleep

Modafinil for Narcolepsy

ABEER J. HANI

> ... as little as a 200-mg daily dose of modafinil is an effective and well-tolerated treatment of EDS [excessive daytime sleepiness] in patients with narcolepsy...
> —The Modafinil for Narcolepsy Study investigators[1]

Research Question: Would the use of either modafinil 200 mg or 400 mg every day safely decrease the excessive daytime sleepiness (EDS) associated with narcolepsy?[1]

Funding: Draxis Health Inc., Mississauga, Ontario, Canada.

Year Study Began: 1995

Year Study Published: 1997

Study Location: 9 different sleep disorder clinics in Canada.

Who Was Studied: 75 patients with confirmed narcolepsy based on criteria of the 1990 international classification of sleep disorders[2] and/or multiple sleep latency testing.

Who Was Excluded: Patients with chronic amphetamine treatment in the last 2 months; EDS attributed to another medical or mental disorder; shift work; a history of head trauma; known hypersensitivity to modafinil; illicit drug use; the use of antipsychotic medication; the use of any medication that might influence sleep (particularly REM sleep) or contribute to EDS, except for anticataplectic medications that were continued in constant dosage; and narcoleptic patients with coexistent, significant sleep apnea (apnea index >10/hour or respiratory disturbance index >20/hour).

How Many Patients: 75

Study Overview: See Figure 29.1 for a summary of the study's design.

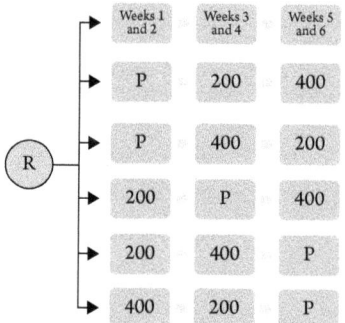

Trial design: R: randomized, P: placebo, 200 = modafinil 200 mg/day, 400 = modafinil 400 mg/day.

Figure 29.1 Summary of the Study's Design.

Study Intervention: Each patient received each of the following treatments during one of the three 2-week periods: placebo, modafinil 200 mg, or modafinil 400 mg in divided doses (morning and noon).

Follow Up: 2 weeks (efficacy data collected during the second week of each 2-week period).

Endpoints: Primary outcome: mean sleep latency on the Maintenance of Wakefulness Test (MWT)[3] (Table 29.1) and the mean number of sleep episodes and periods of severe sleepiness reported in a detailed patient diary. Secondary outcomes: likelihood of falling asleep as measured by the Epworth Sleepiness Scale (ESS)[4] (Table 29.1), as well as tolerance and safety of modafinil.

Table 29.1. TESTS USED TO ASSESS OUTCOME MEASURES IN THE STUDY

Test	Definition/Use in the Study
Maintenance of Wakefulness Test	"[Subjects were asked to try and stay awake while sitting in a comfortable chair. The test] consisted of four test sessions separated by 2 hours, and each session was terminated at minute 40 if no sleep had occurred. Sleep latency was then scored as 40 minutes."[1]
Epworth Sleepiness Scale	"Rate[s] the chances that subjects would doze off or fall asleep when in eight different situations commonly encountered in daily life."[4] Examples include when sitting and reading, watching TV, and as a passenger in a car.

RESULTS

- Modafinil 200 and 400 mg significantly increased the mean sleep latency on the MWT by 40% and 54%, respectively, when compared to placebo, with no significant difference between the two doses (Table 29.2).
- Modafinil at both doses reduced the combined number of daytime sleep episodes and periods of severe sleepiness noted in a detailed patient diary.
- Both modafinil dose levels equally reduced the likelihood of falling asleep as measured by the ESS.
- There were no effects of modafinil on nocturnal sleep initiation, maintenance, or architecture; nor were there any effects on sleep apnea, periodic leg movements, or patients' ability to nap voluntarily during the day, nor with their quantity or quality of nocturnal sleep.
- The only significant adverse effects of modafinil were seen at the 400 mg dose, which was associated with more nausea and nervousness than either placebo or the 200 mg dose.

Table 29.2. SUMMARY OF THE STUDY'S KEY FINDINGS

		MODAFINIL		
Outcome	Placebo	200 mg	400 mg	P Value
Sleep latency (min) using the MWT	11.2 ± 9.8	15.7 ± 12.6	17.2 ± 13.0	< 0.001
% increase in sleep latency compared to placebo		40.4%	53.6%	< 0.001
Patient diary measures: % decrease in severe somnolence compared to placebo		23.9%	25.8%	< 0.01

Criticisms and Limitations: There was no washout period in this study. The validated MWT test was modified ("test consisted of four, not five, test sessions separated by 2 hours, and each session was terminated at minute 40 if no sleep had occurred, rather than at minute 20")[1] with no validation of the modified test method used in this study. Previous medications used to treat narcolepsy were continued, a design that may have confounded the results of this study. There was a short duration of follow-up.

Other Relevant Studies and Information:

- Patients enrolled in this study were followed up further in another study[5] where it was shown again that modafinil at a dose of 330 mg continues to be an effective and well-tolerated drug after 16 weeks of treatment.
- The US Modafinil in Narcolepsy Multicenter Study Group[6,7] also showed that modafinil is an effective treatment for EDS in narcolepsy and has continued efficacy with up to 9 weeks of daily use. Modafinil continued to show a favorable profile for up to 40 weeks of open-label use.
- The practice parameters issued by the American Academy of Sleep Medicine in 2007 for the treatment of narcolepsy and other hypersomnias of central origin cited modafinil as one of the effective treatments for excessive sleepiness associated with narcolepsy.[8]

Summary and Implications: For patients whose narcolepsy is poorly controlled by other stimulants, modafinil is effective and well tolerated. A 200 mg dose has similar efficacy to a 400 mg dose and fewer side effects.

CLINICAL CASE: MODAFINIL FOR NARCOLEPSY

Case History:
A 48-year-old man with a 10-year history of narcolepsy is evaluated for persistent EDS despite the optimization of his amphetamine that was started 1 month ago. Based on the results of this study, how should this patient be treated?

Suggested Answer:
Given the narcolepsy is poorly controlled by amphetamines, a trial of modafinil may be recommended. Given the equal efficacy of the 200 mg versus 400 mg daily dose of modafinil, modafinil 200 mg daily may be prescribed, as the lower dose has fewer adverse effects. Close evaluation and follow-up of this patient using the MWT and the ESS, along with use of a patient diary, may be helpful to better characterize response to modafinil and guide future therapy.

References

1. Broughton RJ, Fleming JA, George CF, et al. Randomized, double-blind, placebo-controlled crossover trial of modafinil in the treatment of excessive daytime sleepiness in narcolepsy. *Neurology*. 1997;49:444–451.
2. Diagnostic Steering Committee; Thorpy M. *International Classification of Sleep Disorders: Diagnostic and Coding Manual*. Rochester, MN: American Sleep Disorders Association; 1990.
3. Mitler MM, Gujavarty KS, Browman CP. Maintenance of wakefulness test: a polysomnographic technique for evaluating treatment efficacy in patients with excessive somnolence. *Electroencephalogr Clin Neurophysiol*. 1982;53:658–661.
4. Johns M. New method for measuring daytime sleepiness: the Epworth Sleepiness Scale. *Sleep*. 1991;14:540–545.
5. Moldofsky H, Broughton RJ, Hill JD. A randomized trial of the long-term, continued efficacy and safety of modafinil in narcolepsy. *Sleep Med*. 2000;1(2):109–116.
6. US Modafinil in Narcolepsy Multicenter Study Group. Randomized trial of modafinil for the treatment of pathological somnolence in narcolepsy. *Ann Neurol*. 1998;43(1):88–97.
7. US Modafinil in Narcolepsy Multicenter Study Group. Randomized trial of modafinil as a treatment for the excessive daytime somnolence of narcolepsy. *Neurology*. 2000;54(5):1166–1175.
8. Morgenthaler TI, Kapur VK, Brown T, et al. Practice parameters for the treatment of narcolepsy and other hypersomnias of central origin. *Sleep*. 2007;30(12):1705–1711.

Continuous Dopamine Agonist for Restless Legs Syndrome

ASHISH L. RANPURA

> ... transdermal delivery of low doses of rotigotine for 24 h per day are more effective than placebo in relieving the symptoms of restless legs syndrome in patients who are moderately to severely affected.
> —TRENKWALDER ET AL.[1]

Research Question: Traditional treatment strategies for restless legs syndrome (RLS) have emphasized evening doses of oral dopaminergic agonists with a focus on alleviating nighttime symptoms. Does 24-hour continuous dopaminergic therapy offer symptomatic and functional benefits to patients with RLS?[1]

Funding: Schwartz Biosciences GmbH, UCB Group (Monheim, Germany).

Year Study Began: 2005

Year Study Published: 2008

Study Location: 49 centers in Austria, Finland, Germany, Italy, the Netherlands, Spain, Sweden, and the United Kingdom.

Who Was Studied: Patients 18–75 years old diagnosed with idiopathic RLS by the four cardinal clinical features defined by the International Restless Legs

Syndrome Study Group (IRLSSG; an overwhelming urge to move the limbs, which is worse at night and negligible in the morning, and triggered by rest and/or sleep, and symptoms which are persistently relieved with movement). Patients were either treatment naïve or were known to be treatment responsive. Further inclusion criteria comprised a baseline sum score of at least 15 on the International Restless Legs Scale (IRLS), which measure RLS severity, and a score of at least 4 for the Clinical Global Impressions (CGI) item 1 assessment (severity of symptoms).

The IRLS score is derived from a short 10-item questionnaire that asks patients about the severity of their RLS symptoms. Responses range from "None" (0 points) to "Very severe" (4 points) on a Likert-type scale, with high scores corresponding to the most severe symptoms. The sum score used in the present study therefore ranges from 0–40, with scores from 0–10 indicative of mild symptoms, 11–20 severe symptoms, and 31–40 very severe symptoms. The questionnaire is a valid subjective measure of patient perceptions, with normally distributed results corresponding well to the functional impacts of the syndrome.[2]

The CGI is a well-established tool to assess a patient's global functioning prior to and after a medical intervention.[3] It is an extremely short, 3-item questionnaire in which a clinician is asked to assess (1) the severity of the patient's disease, (2) the total degree of clinical change relative to baseline, and (3) the efficacy of the target intervention for the patient at hand. The first 2 questions are scored from 1–7, with high scores corresponding to severe illness and clinical deterioration. The third question, that of efficacy, is scored along two dimensions: therapeutic effect (unchanged to marked improvement) and side effects (none to effects that outweigh therapeutic effect), yielding a score from 1–16. The purpose of the CGI scores is to capture a high-level view of a single clinician's overall impression of a medical intervention.

Who Was Excluded: Patients were excluded if they presented with secondary restless legs syndrome. Other exclusion criteria included a current history of sleep disturbances other than RLS (including sleep apnea) and concomitant treatment with neuropharmacologic agents. Patients with central nervous system or peripheral nervous system comorbidities were also excluded. The following were also exclusion criteria: skin hypersensitivity to adhesives or other transdermal preparations; myocardial infarction over the previous 12 months; clinically relevant cardiac, renal, or hepatic dysfunction; arterial peripheral vascular disease; a prolonged QTc interval; symptomatic orthostatic hypotension at screening or baseline; or intake of an investigational drug 28 days before the baseline visit. Pregnant or lactating women, women without effective contraceptive methods, and patients with work-related irregular sleep patterns were also excluded.

How Many Patients: 458

Study Overview: See Figure 30.1 for a summary of the trial design.

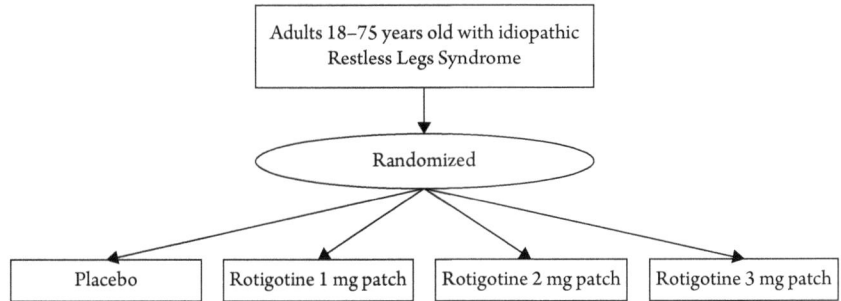

Figure 30.1 Summary of Trial Design.

Study Intervention: The intervention involved a 3-week initiation phase, a 6-month maintenance phase, and a 1-week drug taper. Patients who had been on excluded medications before the trial began had a 4-week washout of prior medications before the initiation phase. During initiation, all patients applied one 5 cm^2 study patch per day in week 1, two such patches in week 2, and finally one 5 cm^2 and one 10 cm^2 patch in week 3 and thereafter. All three rotigotine groups started with a 1 mg daily patch, and were titrated up to their randomized fixed dose in weekly 1 mg steps. If side effects were troubling, back-titration to a lower dose was permitted during the initiation phase only.

During the 6-month maintenance phase, dose adjustments were not made.

Follow-Up: 6 months (at the end of the maintenance phase), with last observation carried forward when necessary.

Endpoints: The two primary outcomes were the IRLS sum score, derived from a patient self-assessment questionnaire, and the CGI item 1 subscore, reflecting an overall clinical assessment of symptom severity. Secondary outcomes included the proportion of IRLS treatment responders (defined as an improvement of >50% in the IRLS score), the proportion of CGI responders (defined as an improvement of >50% in the CGI-1 sub-score), and the proportion with substantial clinical remission of disease (defined as an endpoint IRLS sum score >10). Further secondary measures included changes in the RLS-QoL (quality of life) questionnaire and the RLS-6 severity scale.

A baseline determination of the IRLS and CGI scores was made just prior to the initiation phase. Patients were assessed in the clinic monthly. At the conclusion of the maintenance phase, there followed a final safety assessment.

The RLS-6 scale measures patient perceptions of severity of disease at varying times of day and night. Each question is answered on an 11-point scale, with higher numbers corresponding to more severe symptoms. The scale has been validated for tracking changes in subjective perception of disease over time.[4]

RESULTS

- The highest rate of dropouts occurred amongst the placebo group, mostly due to lack of efficacy. Dropouts in the rotigotine treatment groups were due to adverse events (most commonly application site irritation, nausea, and headache), which were most frequent in the high-dose rotigotine group.
- The mean IRLS sum score, which reflects subjective patient experience of disease, improved from baseline in all 4 groups. The maximum improvement was reached by the end of the 4-week initiation phase, and this effect endured for the full 6-week maintenance phase. Each of the three rotigotine-treated groups had a statistically significant improvement relative to placebo ($P < 0.0001$; see Table 30.1).
- All 3 rotigotine-treated groups had a higher proportion of IRLS- and CGI-defined treatment responders relative to placebo ($P < 0.0001$ for IRLS, $P < 0.005$ for CGI item 1 for all 3 treatment groups compared to placebo). There was no dose-response relationship.
- Subjective quality-of-life scores (RLS-QoS) improved in the rotigotine-treated group in a dose-dependent fashion.
- Daytime symptoms were considered moderate to severe if the baseline RLS-6 score ranged from 5–10. These were considered clinically improved if the score ranged from 0–2 at the end of the trial. Moderate-to-severe daytime symptoms were improved in the majority of rotigotine-treated patients.
- Nearly 20% of patients in the high-dose group dropped out because of intolerable side effects.

Table 30.1. SUMMARY OF THE TRIAL'S KEY FINDINGS

	Placebo	Rotigotine Patch Dosage		
		1 mg	2 mg	3 mg
Mean IRLS change (Standard error)[a]	−8.7 (0.9)	−14.0 (0.8)	−16.4 (1.0)	−16.8 (1.1)
Patients with daytime symptoms at baseline (%)	67/114 (59%)	72/112 (64%)	62/109 (57%)	69/112 (62%)
Patients with resolution of daytime symptoms (%)	20 (30%)	35 (49%)	35 (56%)	40 (58%)

[a] Figures indicate the actual administered dosages, rather than intention-to-treat dosages. All results of the rotigotine groups compared to placebo were significant to $P < 0.0001$.

Criticisms and Limitations: Many patients with RLS do have daytime symptoms, but these are usually quite mild. However, the majority of patients enrolled in the study had moderate-to-severe daytime symptoms in addition to their nighttime symptoms. Since RLS studies have typically excluded patients with significant daytime symptoms, the patient population in this study is different from other study populations, and may have experienced more benefits from continuous dopamine therapy. Placebo effects are known to be very significant in clinical trials for RLS.[5] While rotigotine performed better than placebo, whether continuous dopamine administration offers benefits over more traditional once daily medications is unknown. To date, there are no head-to-head trials to address that question.

Other Relevant Studies and Information:

- The years following the publication of this study have not seen a more widespread use of continuous dopamine agonism for RLS, likely for several reasons. First, the side effects of continuous dopamine agonism are often troubling to patients. Second, the symptoms of RLS are typically mild, and nonpharmacological interventions are often effective. These include limitation of caffeine and tobacco, improved sleep hygiene, and changing the timing of other medications (particularly SSRIs). Finally, a wide range of pharmacological therapies have proven efficacy. Once daily agents may minimize side effects relative to continuous administration formulations like the rotigotine patch, and options include oral dopaminergic agents (pramipexole, ropinirole, levodopa), low-dose benzodiazepines (clonazepam), and anticonvulsants (gabapentin, pregabalin).
- The most recent IRLSSG task force guidelines recommend anticonvulsants or dopamine agonists as first-line agents for the treatment of RLS. There is level A evidence for the use of the rotigotine patch for up to 6 months, and level B evidence of its efficacy up to 5 years. The guidelines suggests that rotigotine is preferable to short-acting dopamine agonists in those patients with more severe daytime symptoms.[6]

Summary and Implications: This study was the first large randomized, double-blind, placebo-controlled trial of continuous dopamine agonism for the treatment of RLS. It demonstrated that treatment with 24-hour rotigotine patches provided significant symptomatic relief within 4 weeks, and that this effect was durable for at least 6 months. These benefits were tempered by dose-dependent side effects including application-site reactions, nausea, and headache. Patients with mild RLS and few daytime symptoms would be better served by conservative management and more traditional short-acting oral agents. However, for patients with disabling symptoms during both day and night, or patients with comorbid movement disorders, continuous transdermal dopaminergic therapy may offer significant relief.

CLINICAL CASE: CONTINUOUS DOPAMINE AGONIST FOR RESTLESS LEGS SYNDROME

Case History:
A 65-year-old right-handed gentleman presents to your clinic with his wife. The couple have been married for decades, but in the last few years they have taken to sleeping apart. The patient's wife states that she can't tolerate the continuous kicking, tossing, and turning movements that her partner makes at night. The patient tells you that he can't stop the feeling of needing to move, and that it's easier for him to sleep on the couch now. When he wakes up in the morning, though, the cushions are scattered over the floor, and the room is a wreck. He states that he usually falls asleep easily, but that he tends to wake up around 3:00 AM and can't fall back asleep. Instead of lying in bed, he starts doing activities like cleaning around the house or surfing the Internet. He has a nap most afternoons and tosses and turns then as well. He doesn't feel excessively sleepy during the daytime, but finds that any time he sits down for a length of time he feels the urge to shift around and move his legs. He drinks 6–8 cups of coffee a day, and takes medications for hypertension and hyperlipidemia.

Laboratory studies, including serum ferritin, are within normal limits. The patient would like to start a medication to help with his symptoms. What do you suggest?

Suggested Answer:
This patient meets the clinical criteria for RLS, most importantly including an urge to move his legs, which is worse at night. His symptoms are having a significant functional impact on his life, so therapy is warranted. You should first suggest that the patient wean himself off of caffeine and improve his sleep hygiene.

Dopamine agonists are the first-line pharmacological agents for RLS. In this patient with prominent daytime symptoms, a continuous agonist like rotigotine would be preferable to a short-acting once daily agonist like ropinirole. He should be followed to assess how his symptoms progress over time.

References

1. Trenkwalder C, Benes H, Poewe W, et al. Efficacy of rotigotine for treatment of moderate-to-severe restless legs syndrome: A randomised, double-blind, placebo-controlled trial. *Lancet Neurol*. 2008;7:595–604
2. The International Restless Legs Syndrome Study Group (Arthur S. Walters MD—Group Organizer and Correspondent). Validation of the International Restless Legs Syndrome Study Group rating scale for restless legs syndrome. *Sleep Medicine*. 2003;4(2):121–132.
3. 028 CGI Clinical Global Impressions. In: Guy W, ed. *ECDEU Assessment Manual for Psychopharmacology*. Rockville, MD: National Institute of Mental Health, 1976: 217–222.
4. Kohnen R, Oertel WH, Stiasny-Kolster K, Benes H, Trenkwalder C. Severity rating of Restless Legs Syndrome: review of ten years experience with the RLS-6 scales in clinical trials. *Sleep*. 2003;26:A342.
5. Fulda S, Wetter TC. Where dopamine meets opioids: a meta-analysis of the placebo effect in RLS treatment studies. *Brain*. 2007;4:902–917.
6. Garcia-Borreguero D, Kohnen R, Silber MH, et al. The long-term treatment of restless legs syndrome/Willis–Ekbom disease: evidence-based guidelines and clinical consensus best practice guidance: a report from the International Restless Legs Syndrome Study Group. *Sleep Medicine*. 2013;14(7):675–684.

SECTION XIII

Spine Disorders

31
Early Surgery for Sciatica

LUIS KOLB

> The 1-year outcomes were similar for patients assigned to early surgery and those assigned to conservative treatment with eventual surgery if needed, but the rates of pain relief and of perceived recovery were faster for those assigned to early surgery.
> —PEUL ET AL.[1]

Research Question: How does early surgery compare with prolonged conservative treatment for patients with severe sciatica?[1]

Funding: Netherlands Organization for Health Research and Development (ZonMW) and the Hoelen Foundation, The Hague.

Year Study Began: November 2002 to February 2005

Year Study Published: 2007

Study Location: Multiple centers in the Netherlands.

Who Was Studied: Patients with 6–12 weeks of severe sciatica. Eligible patients were aged 18–65 years, had a radiographically confirmed disk herniation, and had received a neurologist's diagnosis of an incapacitating lumbosacral radicular syndrome that had lasted from 6–12 weeks.

Who Was Excluded: Patients who presented with cauda equina syndrome, muscle paralysis, insufficient strength to move against gravity, a previous episode of similar symptoms during the prior 12 months, previous spine surgery, bony stenosis, spondylolisthesis, pregnancy, or severe coexisting disease.

How many patients: 283

Study Overview: See Figure 31.1 for a summary of the study design.

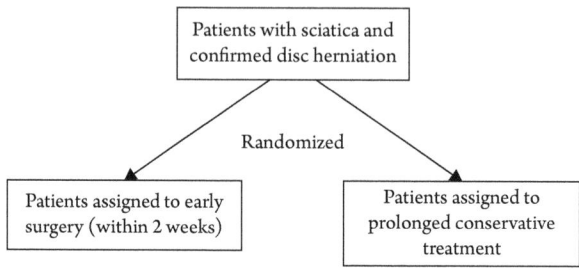

Figure 31.1 Summary of Study Design.

Study Intervention: Patients were randomized to undergoing early surgery or initial prolonged conservative therapy followed by surgery, if needed. Patients who were assigned to early surgery were scheduled to do so within 2 weeks. Open unilateral microdiscectomy was performed. Patients who were assigned to have prolonged conservative therapy continued to do so for an additional 6 months. Surgery was then offered at the 6-month mark to patients who continued to have sciatica symptoms. Patients who had increasing leg pain unresponsive to medication or progressive neurological deficits were offered surgery earlier than 6 months. General practitioners defined conservative treatment, and treatment was mainly aimed at resuming daily activities.

Follow-Up: 1 year.

Endpoints: Primary endpoints were functional disability, intensity of leg pain, and global perceived recovery; and were assessed at 2, 4, 8, 12, 26, 38, and 52 weeks (using the Roland Disability Questionnaire for Sciatica, the 100 mm visual analogue scale [VAS] for leg pain, and the 7-point Likert self-rating scale of global perceived recovery, respectively). Additionally, a repeat neurological examination, functional and economic observational assessments, scores on the Medical Outcomes Study 36-Item Short-Form General Health Survey (SF-36) scale, the Sciatica Frequency and Bothersome Indexes, and a 100 mm VAS for health perception were obtained at 8, 26, and 52 weeks as secondary endpoints.

RESULTS

- Of 141 patients assigned to surgery, 16 recovered before surgery was performed. The remaining 125 patients had surgery within 2 weeks.
- Of the 142 patients assigned to prolonged conservative treatment, 55 underwent surgery during the first year after a median period of 15 weeks due to intractable pain.
- There was no significant difference in disability at 1 year between the two (see Table 31.1).
- There was significant difference between the groups for leg pain, favoring early surgery. After surgery, leg and associated back pain diminished quickly, versus a slower linear recovery in the group receiving initial conservative therapy.
- One year after randomization, there was no significant difference between the groups in the mean scores for any outcome measurement, including leg pain.
- The 55 patients who were assigned to conservative treatment and later underwent surgery had a similar improvement in pain and disability at the 1-year mark compared to the patients who underwent early surgery.
- The median time to recovery was 4 weeks for early surgery, and 12 weeks for conservative management.
- Relief of symptoms was twice as fast among patients with sciatica who were treated with early surgery versus those who were treated with initial prolonged conservative treatment.

Table 31.1. DIFFERENCE BETWEEN CONSERVATIVE TREATMENT AND EARLY SURGERY (95% CI)

	2 weeks	8 weeks	26 weeks	52 weeks
Roland Disability Questionnaire Score	−1.6 (−2.8 to −0.3)	3.1 (1.7 to 4.3)	0.8 (−0.5 to 2.1)	0.4 (−0.9 to 1.7)
VAS score for leg pain	15.7 (11.7 to 19.7)	17.7 (12.3 to 23.1)	6.1 (2.2 to 10)	0 (−4.0 to 4.0)
VAS score for back pain	1.5 (−4.5 to 7.4)	11.3 (5.6 to 17.4)	2.3 (−3.6 to 8.2)	2.3 (−3.6 to 8.2)
Likert score for global perception of recovery	0.4 (0.1 to 0.6)	0.9 (0.6 to 1.2)	0.2 (−.01 to 0.5)	0.2 (−0.1 to 0.4)

NOTE: Negative difference means better outcome with conservative treatment; positive difference means better outcome with surgery.

Criticisms and Limitations: Surgical morbidity was very low (1.6%) and self-limited. Minor criticism has focused on the surgical technique chosen (open unilateral microdiscectomy) instead of newer minimally invasive techniques that could further reduce the time to recovery. Also, the exact timing of recovery could not be precisely determined for each modality, as patients were assessed at predetermined intervals and not continuously. Last, it should be pointed out the focus of the study was on an intention-to-treat analysis, and there was substantial crossover between patients assigned into the conservative group into undergoing surgery. This last effect was reduced by having patients assigned to the early surgery group undergo their procedure within 2 weeks, earlier than prior comparable studies.

Other Relevant Studies and Information:

- Previous studies have demonstrated advantages of surgery relative to conservative management for patients with sciatica in the short term but not in the long term. A landmark randomized clinical trial in 1983 that compared surgery with conservative care (excluding patients with intolerable pain) followed patients for 10 years and found that surgery was superior at the 1-year mark, but by 4 years there was no difference between surgery and conservative treatment.[2]
- More recent studies have conflicting results. One study compared surgery versus conservative treatment and found no differences between the two treatments.[3] An observational cohort study conducted within the same trial included patients who received their preferred treatment. Both groups improved substantially over time, but surgery showed significantly better results for pain and function as compared with the conservative treatment.[4]
- One small trial compared microdiscectomy with conservative treatment in patients with sciatica for 6–12 weeks, and found no significant difference for leg pain, back pain, or subjective disability through the 2 years of follow-up. VAS leg pain scores, however, improved more rapidly in the discectomy group.[5]
- A recent 5-year follow-up from Peul et al. showed no significant difference at 1, 2, and 5 years in disability and pain between patients allocated to either early surgery or 6 months of prolonged conservative care. In that study, 8% never showed recovery, while 23% of all patients had ongoing complaints, which fluctuated over time, irrespective of treatment. Of note, 46% of patients assigned to

conservative therapy needed surgery after a few months of prolonged sciatica.[6]

Summary and Implications: For patients with severe sciatica that persists beyond 6–12 weeks, surgery leads to faster improvements in pain; however, after 1 year of follow-up the two approaches have similar outcomes. Although in many countries clinical guidelines are available for the management of nonspecific low back pain, this is not the case for sciatica. It is generally recommended to refer patients for surgical evaluation in cases of intractable radicular pain, or for pain that does not improve after 6–8 weeks of conservative care.

CLINICAL CASE: PATIENT WITH SCIATICA

Case History:
A 56-year-old woman presents to clinic with several weeks of severe L5 radicular pain of the right leg. She works as a teacher, and states that the pain is affecting her job and has caused her to miss several days of work. She is sent for 6 weeks of pain control and physical therapy, and returns to clinic without improvement in her symptoms. Her imaging shows a right-sided L5 herniated disc abutting the nerve root.

How should you advise this patient about her options?

Suggested Answer:
Based on the current evidence, this patient has the choice to continue conservative treatment or undergo surgery with microdiscectomy.

Continuing conservative therapy has a good chance of relieving her symptoms, but there is still a chance of needing surgery to relieve her symptoms at a later date.

Delaying surgery in the hopes her symptoms improve does not hurt her chances of a complete recovery by 1 year.

Early surgery provides the benefit of quicker relief of pain and faster recovery. If the patient is not able to cope with the leg pain, finds the natural course to recovery (6–12 months) slow, or wants to minimize her time to recovery, she might opt for early surgery. Otherwise, she might choose to delay surgery and see if her symptoms improve or resolve with conservative methods. If the symptoms worsen or do not improve, she can choose surgery at a later date without affecting her chances to recover.

References

1. Peul WC, van Houwelingen HC, van den Hout WB, et al. Surgery versus prolonged conservative treatment for sciatica. *N Engl J Med.* 2007;356:2245–2256. doi:10.1056/NEJMoa064039.
2. Weber H. Lumbar disc herniation. A controlled, prospective study with ten years of observation. *Spine.* 1983;8(2):131–140.
3. Weinstein JN, Tosteson TD, Lurie JD, et al. Surgical vs nonoperative treatment for lumbar disk herniation: the Spine Patient Outcomes Research Trial (SPORT): a randomized trial. *JAMA.* 2006;296(20);2441–2450. doi:10.1001/jama.296.20.2441.
4. Weinstein JN, Lurie JD, Tosteson TD, et al. Surgical vs nonoperative treatment for lumbar disk herniation: the Spine Patient Outcomes Research Trial (SPORT) observational cohort. *JAMA.* 2006;296(20):2451–2459. doi:10.1001/jama.296.20.2451.
5. Osterman H, Seitsalo S, Karppinen J, Malmivaara A. Effectiveness of microdiscectomy for lumbar disc herniation: a randomized controlled trial with 2 years of follow-up. *Spine.* 2006;31(21):2409–2414. doi:10.1097/01.brs.0000239178.08796.52.
6. Lequin MB, Verbaan D, Jacobs WCH, et al. Surgery versus prolonged conservative treatment for sciatica: 5-year results of a randomised controlled trial. *BMJ Open.* 2013;3:e002534. doi:10.1136/bmjopen-2012-002534.

Surgery for Lumbar Degenerative Spondylolisthesis
The SPORT Trial

RYAN A. GRANT

... [P]atients with degenerative spondylolisthesis and spinal stenosis treated surgically showed substantially greater improvement in pain and function during a period of 2 years than patients treated nonsurgically.
—THE SPORT INVESTIGATORS[1]

Research Question: Is surgery effective for lumbar degenerative spondylolisthesis (i.e., slipping forward of one lumbar vertebra on another) with spinal stenosis compared to nonsurgical treatment?[1]

Funding: National Institute of Arthritis and Musculoskeletal and Skin Diseases (NIAMS), NIH, National Institute of Occupational Safety and Health, Centers for Disease Control and Prevention, and the Multidisciplinary Clinical Research Center in Musculoskeletal Diseases.

Year Study Began: 2000

Year Study Published: 2007

Study Location: 13 medical centers in United States.

Who Was Studied: Patients ≥18 years old were eligible if they had 12 weeks of neurogenic claudication or lower extremity radiculopathy with imaging-confirmed degenerative lumbar spondylolisthesis on standing lateral radiographs. Most of the degenerative slips were at L4/L5.

Who Was Excluded: Patients with <12 weeks of symptoms, patients with spondylolysis (e.g., stress fracture of a lumbar vertebra) or isthmic spondylolisthesis (e.g., stress fracture leading to vertebra slippage); nonsurgical candidates; and patients who presented with inadequate nonsurgical treatment, fractures, infections, deformity, and/or cancer.

How Many Patients: 304 patients in a randomized cohort and 303 in an observational cohort.

Study Overview: See Figure 32.1 for a summary of the trial's design.

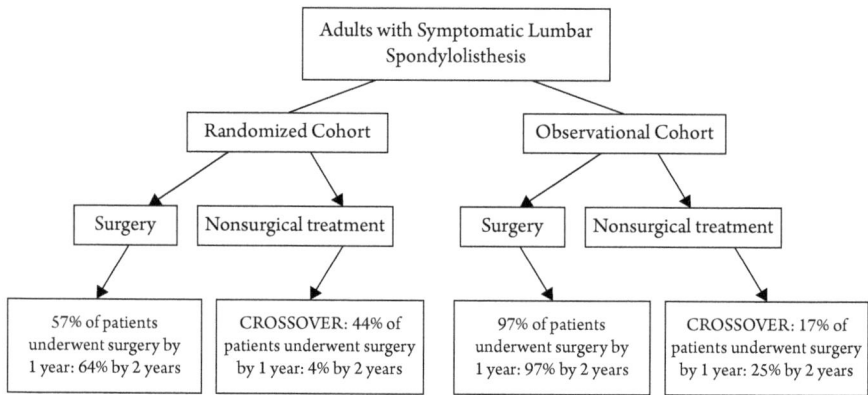

Figure 32.1 Summary of SPORT's Design.

Study Intervention: The randomized cohort received either surgical decompression or nonsurgical care including at least physical therapy, instructions for exercising at home, and nonsteroidal anti-inflammatory agents. The patients in the observational cohort chose either surgical decompression or conservative therapy and were followed. Surgery consisted of standard decompressive laminectomy with or without a single-level fusion (iliac crest bone grafting with or without posterior pedicle-screw instrumentation).

Follow-Up: 2 years.

Endpoints: Primary outcome measures were the Medical Outcomes Study 36-Item Short-Form General Health Survey (SF-36) bodily pain and physical function scores[2] (100-point scale, with higher scores = less severe symptoms) and the modified Oswestry Disability Index[3] (100-point scale, with lower scores = less severe symptoms) at 6 weeks, 3 months, 6 months, 1 year, and 2 years. Secondary outcomes included subjective improvement, patient satisfaction with current symptoms, the Stenosis Bothersomeness Index[4,5] (24-point scale, with lower scores = less severe symptoms), and the Low Back Pain Bothersomeness Scale[6] (6-point scale, with lower scores = less severe symptoms).

RESULTS

- Intention-to-treat analysis of the randomized cohort showed no significant advantage for surgery over nonsurgical care for primary outcomes; however, this is severely limited by nonadherence to the assigned treatment. The crossover rate was approximately 40% in both directions; specifically, 49% of patients assigned conservative management underwent surgery (see Table 32.1).
- Thus, analysis for as-treated effects was completed, and for combined cohorts it demonstrated that surgery was significantly superior to nonsurgical treatment in relieving neurogenic claudication/radiculopathy and improving function (all primary and secondary outcomes). Lower back pain was improved with surgery, but not as significantly as other symptoms.
- These effects were seen as early as 6 weeks postintervention and persisted for over 2 years. With regard to the treatment effect attributable to surgery, the difference between the as-treated surgical and nonsurgical groups was 18.1 points for bodily pain for the SF-36 bodily pain score, 18.3 points for the SF-36 physical function score, and –16.7 points for the Oswestry Disability Index.
- Surgical complications were rare, with significant injury in <1% of patients (i.e., vascular injury). The most common complication was a dural tear resulting in a cerebrospinal fluid leak (CSF) in 10% of the patients.
- The reoperation rate at 2 years was 12%, due to combinations of hardware complications, infections, and CSF leaks, as well as recurrent stenosis and progressive listhesis.
- Conversely, the nonsurgical group only had moderate improvement with time (SF-36 function improved by 11.7 points for SF-36 bodily pain, 8.3 points for SF-36 physical function, and –7.5 points for the Oswestry Disability Index).

Table 32.1. SUMMARY OF SPORT's KEY FINDINGS: COMBINED AS-TREATED RANDOMIZED AND OBSERVATIONAL COHORTS

Primary Outcomes	3 MONTHS			1 YEAR			2 YEARS		
	Nonsurgical	Surgical	P Value	Nonsurgical	Surgical	P Value	Nonsurgical	Surgical	P Value
SF-36 change									
Bodily Pain	10.3	28.1	<0.001	12.7	31.5	<0.001	11.7	29.9	<0.001
Function	7.6	21.5	<0.001	9.6	29.0	<0.001	8.3	26.6	<0.001
Oswestry change	−6.2	−20.8	<0.001	−7.5	−25.4	<0.001	−7.5	−24.2	<0.001

Criticisms and Limitations: There was lack of standardization of the interventions in each cohort limiting the internal/external validity as well as overall generalizability. That is, no direct level 1 conclusion regarding the effect of surgery and a specific nonsurgical treatment can be gathered from this trial. Specifically, surgical fusion and surgical decompression were lumped together, not allowing readers to know if fusion is superior. Similarly, the efficacy of nonsurgical treatments compared with a specific surgical intervention also cannot be known. For example, the nonsurgical group received heterogeneous treatments including physical therapy, epidural injections, chiropractic treatment, anti-inflammatory agents, and opioid analgesics, among other nonsurgical interventions,[7] whereas the surgical group underwent decompression with or without fusion, each adding a complexity of variability and limiting the generalizability of the results.[8] The intention-to-treat cohort had a very high crossover rate (49%), with marked nonadherence to randomization, limiting the power to demonstrate a treatment effect. Only the as-treated groups had the power to demonstrate a treatment effect; they are confounded by lack of randomization, but do provide good level 2 evidence.

Other Relevant Studies and Information:

- Four-year outcome data from the SPORT trial continues to demonstrate that as-treated patients with degenerative spondylolisthesis and associated spinal stenosis treated surgically have substantially greater pain relief and improvement in function.[9]
- Similarly, surgery for spinal stenosis without spondylolisthesis results in significantly better pain relief and improvement in function.[10]
- Substantial improvement occurs in patients with symptomatic lumbar degenerative disease, including spondylolisthesis, of at least 12 weeks when treated surgically.[11]
- The Maine Lumbar Spine Study demonstrated that patients with severe lumbar spinal stenosis who were treated surgically had greater improvement than patients treated nonsurgically at 1 year,[6] as well as at 4 years.[12] However, the effect became less significant 8–10 years out.[13]

- Conversely, Cochrane Reviews up to the year 2005 have found no evidence for the effectiveness of surgical intervention for spondylosis compared to nonsurgical management given a lack of randomized controlled trials.[14]
- Taking into account all of the available evidence, the North American Spine Society (NASS)—the largest spine society in the United States—released updated evidence-based clinical guidelines for multidisciplinary spine care in 2014 and recommend that "direct *surgical decompression* [can] be considered for the treatment of patients with symptomatic spinal stenosis associated with low grade degenerative lumbar spondylolisthesis whose symptoms have been recalcitrant to a trial of medical/interventional treatment."[15] NASS notes that this is based on poor evidence with no randomized controlled trials.
- However, there is level 2 evidence[16] that surgical decompression with fusion is superior to decompression alone, which is something the SPORT trial did not assess given that all types of surgery were combined. Additionally, based on level 2 evidence, NASS goes on to state that "surgical decompression with fusion, with or without instrumentation, is suggested to improve the functional outcomes of single-level degenerative spondylolisthesis compared to medical/interventional treatment alone."[15]

Summary and Implications: In this trial, patients with persistent neurogenic claudication and/or lumbar radiculopathy from degenerative spondylolisthesis with spinal stenosis treated surgically had substantially greater improvement in pain and function, as well as satisfaction, that persisted long term compared to nonoperative treatments. Based on all the evidence, including this study, guidelines recommend that surgery can be considered for patients with symptomatic spinal stenosis associated with low-grade degenerative lumbar spondylolisthesis if conservative measures have proven ineffective.

CLINICAL CASE: SURGERY FOR LUMBAR DEGENERATIVE SPONDYLOLISTHESIS

Case History:
A 63-year-old male with several years of chronic lower back pain, neurogenic claudication, and an L4 radiculopathy of the right leg presents for evaluation. The symptoms are greatly affecting his ability to perform his job as a building contractor. He has tried physical therapy, with only modest results, but not any other conservative measure. He is interested in surgery, but unsure about the potential success, and scared about potential complications. His imaging demonstrates a grade I spondylolisthesis at L4/L5 with moderate associated spinal stenosis.

Suggested Answer:
The SPORT trial demonstrates that individuals with 12 weeks of neurogenic claudication or lower extremity radiculopathy from lumbar spondylolisthesis with stenosis will most likely have a better improvement in pain and function if treated surgically. However, if treated nonsurgically, the SPORT trial demonstrates that it is expected that the patient will improve, or at minimum remain stable, without surgical intervention. The trial unfortunately cannot speak to the timing of surgery in comparison to nonsurgical management, the degree of spondylolisthesis and stenosis requiring surgery, and whether a fusion should be performed if surgery is pursued. Thus, each case has to be considered on an individual basis, with clear goal-directed therapy recommended to each patient.

References

1. Weinstein JN, Lurie JD, Tosteson TD, et al. Surgical versus nonsurgical treatment for lumbar degenerative spondylolisthesis. *N Engl J Med*. 2007;356(22):2257–2270.
2. McHorney CA, Ware JE Jr, Lu JF, Sherbourne CD. The MOS 36-item Short-Form Health Survey (SF-36): III. Tests of data quality, scaling assumptions, and reliability across diverse patient groups. *Medical Care*. 1994;32(1):40–66.
3. Daltroy LH, Cats-Baril WL, Katz JN, Fossel AH, Liang MH. The North American Spine Society Lumbar Spine Outcome Assessment Instrument: reliability and validity tests. *Spine*. 1996;21(6):741–749.
4. Patrick DL, Deyo RA, Atlas SJ, Singer DE, Chapin A, Keller RB. Assessing health-related quality of life in patients with sciatica. *Spine*. 1995;20(17):1899–1908; discussion 1909.

5. Atlas SJ, Deyo RA, Patrick DL, Convery K, Keller RB, Singer DE. The Quebec Task Force classification for spinal disorders and the severity, treatment, and outcomes of sciatica and lumbar spinal stenosis. *Spine*. 1996;21(24):2885–2892.
6. Atlas SJ, Deyo RA, Keller RB, et al. The Maine Lumbar Spine Study, Part III. 1-year outcomes of surgical and nonsurgical management of lumbar spinal stenosis. *Spine*. 1996;21(15):1787–1794; discussion 1794–1785.
7. Birkmeyer NJ, Weinstein JN, Tosteson AN, et al. Design of the Spine Patient Outcomes Research Trial (SPORT). *Spine*. 2002;27(12):1361–1372.
8. da Costa BR, Johnston BC. Surgical versus nonsurgical treatment for back pain. *N Engl J Med*. 2007;357(12):1255; author reply 1255–1256.
9. Weinstein JN, Lurie JD, Tosteson TD, et al. Surgical compared with nonoperative treatment for lumbar degenerative spondylolisthesis. Four-year results in the Spine Patient Outcomes Research Trial (SPORT) randomized and observational cohorts. *J Bone Joint Surg Am*. 2009;91(6):1295–1304.
10. Weinstein JN, Tosteson TD, Lurie JD, et al. Surgical versus nonsurgical therapy for lumbar spinal stenosis. *N Engl J Med*. 2008;358(8):794–810.
11. Carreon LY, Glassman SD, Howard J. Fusion and nonsurgical treatment for symptomatic lumbar degenerative disease: a systematic review of Oswestry Disability Index and MOS Short Form-36 outcomes. *Spine J*. 2008;8(5):747–755.
12. Atlas SJ, Keller RB, Robson D, Deyo RA, Singer DE. Surgical and nonsurgical management of lumbar spinal stenosis: four-year outcomes from the maine lumbar spine study. *Spine*. 2000;25(5):556–562.
13. Atlas SJ, Keller RB, Wu YA, Deyo RA, Singer DE. Long-term outcomes of surgical and nonsurgical management of lumbar spinal stenosis: 8 to 10 year results from the Maine Lumbar Spine Study. *Spine*. 2005;30(8):936–943.
14. Gibson JN, Waddell G, Grant IC. Surgery for degenerative lumbar spondylosis. *Cochrane Database Syst Rev*. 2000(3):Cd001352.
15. North American Spine Society (NASS) *Diagnosis and Treatment of Degenerative Spondylolisthesis*. 2nd ed. Burr Ridge, IL: North American Spine Society; 2014). https://www.spine.org/Portals/0/Documents/ResearchClinicalCare/Guidelines/Spondylolisthesis.pdf.
16. Liang L, Jiang WM, Li XF, Wang H. Effect of fusion following decompression for lumbar spinal stenosis: a meta-analysis and systematic review. *Int J Clin Exp Med*. 2015;8(9):14615–14624.

Steroids versus No Steroids for Acute Spinal Cord Injury
The NASCIS II Trial
SACIT BULENT OMAY

> [Contrary to NASCIS II,] administration of methylprednisolone (MP) for the treatment of acute spinal cord injury (SCI) is not recommended . . . (American Association of Neurological Surgeons / Congress of Neurological Surgeons (AANS/CNS) Joint Guidelines Committee).
> —Hurlbert et al.[1]

Research Question: Animal studies indicate that high-dose methylprednisolone and naloxone are both potentially beneficial in acute spinal-cord injury, but are they effective in humans?[2]

Funding: Supported by a grant (NS-15078) from the National Institute of Neurological Disorders and Stroke. The study drugs and placebos were provided by the Upjohn Corporation (methylprednisolone) and the DuPont Corporation (naloxone).

Year Study Began: 1985

Year Study Published: 1990

Study Location: 10 sites in the United States.

Who Was Studied: Patients with acute (within 12 hours) spinal-cord injury. Eligible patients were those who had a spinal-cord injury diagnosed by a physician associated with the study, who consented to participate, and who were randomized within 12 hours of their injury.

Who Was Excluded: Ineligible patients were those with involvement of the nerve root or cauda equina only, gunshot wounds, or life-threatening morbidity; those who were pregnant, addicted to narcotics, receiving maintenance steroids for other reasons, or aged <13 years; those who had received more than 100 mg of methylprednisolone or its equivalent, or 1 mg of naloxone, before admission to the center; and those in whom follow-up would be difficult.

How Many Patients: 487

Study Overview: See Figure 33.1 for a summary of the study design.

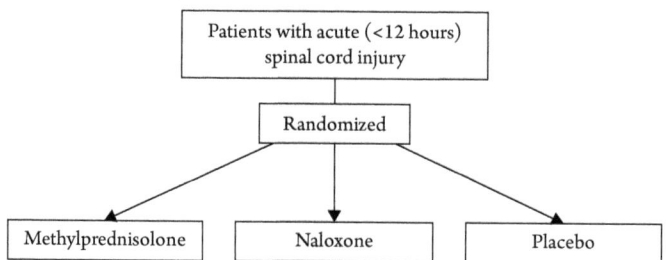

Figure 33.1 Summary of NASCIS II Design.

Study Intervention: After determining a patient's eligibility, the patients were randomized and received one of the 3 protocols. Patients in the methylprednisolone group received a 30 mg/kg bolus, then 5.4 mg/kg/hr for 23 hours intravenously. Patients in the naloxone group received a 5.4 mg/kg bolus, then 4.0 mg/kg/hr for 23 hours intravenously. The placebo group received an intravenous placebo as bolus followed by an infusion as well.

Follow-Up: 6 months (1 year with the follow-up study).[3]

Endpoints: The primary endpoint was a change in neurologic function between baseline and the follow-up examinations performed at 6 weeks and 6 months after injury using categorical and score-type scales to assess motor function, pinprick sensation, and light touch sensation (see Table 33.1).

Table 33.1. Summary of "Assessment of Neurologic Function"

Modality	Complete/Incomplete	Expanded Neurologic Score	Categorical
Pinprick and Light Touch	Yes/No	Absent (1) Decreased (2) Normal (3) 29 segments from C2 to S5 tested, with possible scores ranging from 29 to 87 for each sensory modality	Analgesic & anesthetic above T1 Analgesic & anesthetic below T1 Hypalgesic & hypesthesic above T1 Hypalgesic & hypesthesic below T1 Normal
Motor Function	Yes/No	No contraction (0) Reduced contraction (1) Movement without antigravity (2) Movement with antigravity (3) Movement against resistance (4) Normal function (5) Scored for 14 muscle segments, with possible score ranging from zero to 70	Quadriplegic Quadriparetic Paraparetic Normal

Adapted from Bracken MB, Shepard MJ, Collins WF, et al. A randomized, controlled trial of methylprednisolone or naloxone in the treatment of acute spinal-cord injury. Results of the Second National Acute Spinal Cord Injury Study. *N Engl J Med.* 1990;322(20):1405–1411.

RESULTS

- After 6 months, the patients who were treated with methylprednisolone within 8 hours of their injury had significant improvement, versus those given placebo (see Table 33.2).
- The benefit from methylprednisolone was seen in patients whose injuries were initially evaluated as neurologically complete, as well as in those believed to have incomplete lesions.
- The patients treated with naloxone at any time point, or with methylprednisolone more than 8 hours after their injury, did not differ in their neurologic outcomes from those given placebo.
- Mortality and major morbidity were similar in all three groups.

Table 33.2. SUMMARY OF RESULTS WITHIN 8 HOURS OF INJURY

Drug	CHANGE SCORE		
	Motor Function	Sensation Pinprick	Sensation Touch
Methylprednisolone	16.0 ($P = 0.03$)	11.4 ($P = 0.02$)	8.9 ($P = 0.03$)
Placebo	11.2	6.6	4.3

Criticisms and Limitations: The main criticism of this study was that improvement in motor and sensory change scores at 6 months in patients given methylprednisolone within 8 hours of injury was revealed in post-hoc analyses[1] (patients were not initially stratified and randomized using "within 8 hours of injury" as a criterion). The NASCIS investigators reported motor and sensation "change" scores, reporting on change in the exam scores, not true measures of improvement in motor or sensory functions. They chose to report on right-side-of-body scores only, not the left side of the body or whole body motor and sensory measurements, as only the right side of the body was positive for change in motor or sensory scores. These particular findings were identified in a post-hoc analysis of only 62 methylprednisolone patients, compared to only 65 placebo patients, not the entire study cohort (complete SCI: 45 methylprednisolone vs. 43 placebo patients; incomplete SCI: 17 methylprednisolone vs. 12 placebo patients). Other criticisms were related to how the 8 hour cutoff was assigned, weakness in control groups, and inadequate use of standardized functional outcome tests.[4-6] As a consequence, NASCIS II results are now perceived as class III medical evidence.[1]

Other Relevant Studies and Information: The results of NASCIS II were not supported by other studies that followed it. The prospective blinded randomized controlled trials done in an effort to reveal the effect of steroids in acute spinal cord injury have shown no class I or class II medical evidence for beneficial effect.[2,7-9] Harmful side effects of methylprednisolone administration in the setting of acute SCI have been reported as significant in class I studies.[8-10] The American Association of Neurological Surgeons/Congress of Neurological Surgeons (AANS/CNS) performed an exhaustive medical evidence–based review on this subject. Their published guideline, "Pharmacological Therapy for Acute Spinal Cord Injury," does not support administration of methylprednisolone in the treatment of acute cervical spinal cord injury, and in fact recommends against its use.[1]

Summary and Implications: NASCIS II failed to produce class I or II medical evidence for use of methylprednisolone in the setting of acute spinal cord injury. Furthermore, other studies have not shown evidence to support the use of methylprednisolone in the setting of acute spinal cord injury and have revealed potential complications related to its use. Therefore current clinical guidelines do not recommend use of methylprednisolone in the setting of acute spinal cord injury as the NASCIS II trial initially suggested.

CLINICAL CASE: USE OF METHYLPREDNISOLONE IN ACUTE SPINAL CORD INJURY

Case History:
A 25-year-old male is brought to the emergency room 45 minutes after a motorcycle accident. The patient was found to be unconscious at the scene and was intubated by emergency personnel. A cervical collar was placed at the site, and patient was transferred with strict spine precautions.

On examination, the patient's vital signs are significant for hypotension. He did not have any motor response to noxious stimuli in his lower extremities.

CT of the head was within normal limits. CT of the spine revealed a burst fracture of T3 with severe mass effect on the spinal cord.

Based on the results of NASCIS II, should you treat this patient with methylprednisolone?

Suggested Answer:
The patient is experiencing an acute spinal cord injury with paraplegia and likely spinal shock. He is within the 8-hour window. Based purely on NASCIS II, he should have received methylprednisolone, but our current data reveals that this will fail to improve the outcome, and will expose the patient to complications of high-dose steroids.

References

1. Hurlbert RJ, Hadley MN, Walters BC, et al. Pharmacological therapy for acute spinal cord injury. *Neurosurg.* 2013;72(suppl 2):93–105. doi:1227/NEU.0b013e31827765c6.
2. Bracken MB, Shepard MJ, Collins WF, et al. A randomized, controlled trial of methylprednisolone or naloxone in the treatment of acute spinal-cord injury. Results of the Second National Acute Spinal Cord Injury Study. *N Engl J Med.* 1990;322(20):1405–1411.
3. Bracken MB, Shepard MJ, Collins WF Jr, et al. Methylprednisolone or naloxone treatment after acute spinal cord injury: 1-year follow-up data. Results of the second National Acute Spinal Cord Injury Study. *J Neurosurg.* 1992;76(1):23–31.

4. Hurlbert RJ. Methylprednisolone for acute spinal cord injury: an inappropriate standard of care. *J Neurosurg.* 2000;93(suppl 1):1–7.
5. Short DJ, El Masry WS, Jones PW. High-dose methylprednisolone in the management of acute spinal cord injury—a systematic review from a clinical perspective. *Spinal Cord.* 2000;38:273–286.
6. Coleman WP, Benzel D, Cahill DW, et al. A critical appraisal of the reporting of the National Acute Spinal Cord Injury Studies (II and III) of methylprednisolone in acute spinal cord injury. *J Spinal Disord.* 2000;13:185–199.
7. Bracken MB, Collins WF, Freeman DF, et al. Efficacy of methylprednisolone in acute spinal cord injury. *JAMA.* 1984;251(1):45–52.
8. Bracken MB, Shepard MJ, Holford TR, et al. Administration of methylprednisolone for 24 or 48 hours or tirilazad mesylate for 48 hours in the treatment of acute spinal cord injury. Results of the Third National Acute Spinal Cord Injury Randomized Controlled Trial. National Acute Spinal Cord Injury Study. *JAMA.* 1997;277(20):1597–1604.
9. Pointillart V, Petitjean ME, Wiart L, et al. Pharmacological therapy of spinal cord injury during the acute phase. *Spinal Cord.* 2000;38(2):71–76.
10. Matsumoto T, Tamaki T, Kawakami M, Yoshida M, Ando M, Yamada H. Early complications of high-dose methylprednisolone sodium succinate treatment in the follow-up of acute cervical spinal cord injury. *Spine (Phila Pa 1976).* 2001;26(4):426–430.

SECTION XIV

Vascular Neurology

IV Thrombolysis 3 Hours after an Acute Ischemic Stroke

The NINDS Trial

HARDIK P. AMIN

> ... treatment with intravenous t-PA within three hours of the onset of ischemic stroke improved clinical outcome at three months ...
> —MARLER ET AL.[1]

Research Question: Does the use of intravenous tissue plasminogen activator (t-PA) to treat acute ischemic stroke improve neurologic outcomes if given within 3 hours of symptom onset?[1]

Funding: National Institute of Neurological Disorders and Stroke.

Year Study Began: 1991

Year Study Published: 1995

Study Location: 8 U.S. centers.

Who Was Studied: This trial evaluated patients with acute ischemic stroke or stroke symptoms with a clearly defined time of onset, as well as a deficit measurable on the National Institutes of Health Stroke Scale (NIHSS). A baseline computed tomography (CT) scan ruling out acute intracranial hemorrhage (ICH) was performed on all patients.

Who Was Excluded: "Patients with evidence of acute ICH on CT scan or prior history of ICH; stroke or serious head trauma within the preceding three months; major surgery within the preceding 14 days; systolic blood pressure above 185 mm Hg or diastolic blood pressure above 110 mm Hg; required aggressive treatment to reduce blood pressure to specified limits; rapidly improving or minor symptoms; symptoms suggestive of subarachnoid hemorrhage; gastrointestinal hemorrhage or urinary tract hemorrhage within the previous 21 days; arterial puncture at noncompressible site within the previous 7 days; taking anticoagulants or who had received heparin within the 48 hours preceding the onset of stroke and had an elevated partial thromboplastin time or those with prothrombin times greater than 15 seconds; platelet counts below 100,000 per cubic millimeter; glucose concentrations below 50 mg per deciliter or above 400 mg per deciliter; and who had a seizure at the onset of stroke."[1]

How Many Patients: 624

Study Overview: See Figure 34.1 for a summary of the study design.

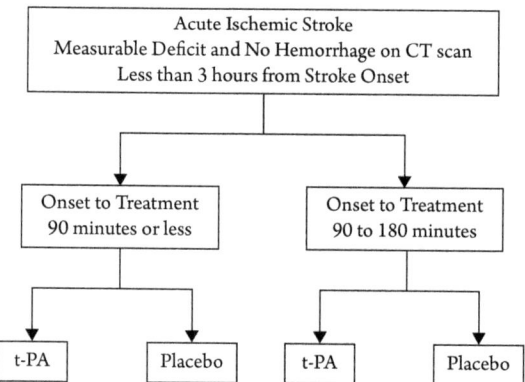

Figure 34.1 Summary of NINDS t-PA Stroke Study Design for Part 1 and Part 2 Trials.

- Part 1 Trial: Tested t-PA clinical activity, defined as complete resolution of the neurological deficit or an improvement from baseline NIHSS by ≥4 points 24 hours after the onset of stroke. Groups were subdivided by time from symptom onset to t-PA administration (0–90 minutes, 91–180 minutes, 0–180 minutes). 291 patients.
- Part 2 Trial: Investigated benefits of t-PA at 90 days postadministration, measured by a global test statistic that used scores on 4 scales: Barthel Index, modified Rankin Scale (mRS), Glasgow Outcome Scale (GOS), and the NIHSS. 333 patients.

Study Intervention: Patients in the t-PA group received 0.9 mg/kg up to maximum 90 mg; 10% as a bolus, then the remaining 90% as a 60-minute infusion. Patients in the placebo groups received intravenous placebo. Treatment with anticoagulants or antiplatelet agents was prohibited for 24 hours posttreatment.

Follow-Up: 90 days.

Endpoints: Primary outcome: Part 1: Complete resolution of neurologic benefit or improvement from baseline NIHSS by >4 points at 24 hours. Part 2: Global assessment at 90 days using the 4 outcome measures listed above to determine favorable outcome (minimal or no significant deficit or disability).

RESULTS

- Part 1 Trial: No statistically significant difference in 4-point NIHSS improvement between the group given t-PA and that given placebo at 24 hours.
- Part 2 Trial: See Table 34.1. In those treated with t-PA, the odds ratio for a favorable outcome represented a 12% absolute increase in the number of patients with minimal or no disability at 3 months, as well as an 11% absolute increase in the number of patients with an NIHSS score of 0 or 1. This benefit was not associated with increased mortality.
- For the t-PA group, 6.4% of patients experienced symptomatic ICH within 36 hours of stroke onset, as opposed to 0.6% in the placebo group ($P < 0.001$).

Table 34.1. OUTCOME AT 90 DAYS IN PART 2 OF THE STUDY, IN TERMS OF PERCENTAGE OF PATIENTS[a]

NIHSS	Placebo	t-PA	Barthel Index	Placebo	t-PA
0–1	20	31	95–100	38	50
2–8	32	30	55–90	23	16
>9	27	22	0–50	18	17
Death	21	17	Death	21	17

mRS[b]	Placebo	t-PA	GOS[c]	Placebo	t-PA
0–1	26	39	1	32	44
2–3	25	21	2	22	17
4–5	27	23	3–4	25	22
Death	21	17	Death	21	17

[a] Of note, lower scores on the NIHSS, mRS, and GOS indicate better outcome, whereas the opposite is true for the Barthel Index.
[b] mRS = Modified Rankin Scale (see Table 35.1 in Chapter 35).
[c] GOS = Glasgow Outcome Scale (see Table 8.1 in Chapter 8).

Criticisms and Limitations: Some follow-up studies documented higher and lower hemorrhage and mortality rates than the NINDS Part 1 and Part 2 trial results, and attributed these rates to the degree of protocol deviations.[2-4] The potential benefit of early treatment (<90 minutes) was not apparent in the initial publication.

Other Relevant Studies and Information:

- The ECASS III trial established that thrombolysis with intravenous alteplase given up to 4.5 hours after the onset of stroke symptoms is modestly efficacious.
- Multiple studies concluded that patients treated within the first 1.5 hours are most likely to have good outcomes.[5,6]
- A 2013 American College of Emergency Physicians guideline finds level A evidence that "in order to improve functional outcomes, IV t-PA should be offered to acute ischemic stroke patients who meet National Institute of Neurological Disorders and Stroke (NINDS) inclusion/exclusion criteria and can be treated within 3 hours after symptom onset."[7]

Summary and Implications: This was the first trial to establish efficacy for intravenous thrombolysis treatment for ischemic stroke with improved clinical outcomes at 3 months. This study provided neurologists with a proven form of treatment for acute ischemic stroke, and reinforced the urgency in which acute stroke cases need to be evaluated and treated.

CLINICAL CASE: IV T-PA FOR ACUTE ISCHEMIC STROKE WITHIN 3 HOURS OF ONSET

Case History:
A 65-year-old male with a history of hypertension, hyperlipidemia, diabetes, and coronary heart disease status post CABG 10 days ago presents to the emergency department with acute onset of left-sided weakness and slurred speech. His wife noticed his sudden change about 1 hour prior to presentation. A noncontrast head CT did not show any acute abnormalities. His NIHSS is 7 for a left facial droop, left arm and leg weakness, and moderate dysarthria.

He has a 30-pack-year smoking history, and occasionally drinks alcohol. His medications include aspirin 325 mg, lisinopril 10 mg, metformin 500 mg twice daily, and simvastatin 40 mg.

Based on the results of this trial, is this patient a candidate for intravenous t-PA?

Suggested Answer:
The trial excluded stroke patients with major surgery (i.e. CABG) within 2 weeks of presentation. This is due to probable increased risk of bleeding at the surgical site. For this reason, this patient would not be a candidate for intravenous t-PA. Antiplatelet use is not a contraindication for t-PA.

References

1. Tissue plasminogen activator for acute ischemic stroke. The National Institute of Neurological Disorders and Stroke rt-PA Stroke Study Group. *N Engl J Med.* 1995;333(24):1581–1587.
2. Lopez-Yunez AM, Bruno A, Williams LS, Yilmaz E, Zurrú C, Biller J. Protocol violations in community-based rT-PA stroke treatment are associated with symptomatic intracerebral hemorrhage. *Stroke.* 2001;32(1):12–16.
3. Bravata DM, Kim N, Concato J, Krumholz HM, Brass LM. Thrombolysis for acute stroke in routine clinical practice. *Arch Intern Med.* 2002;162(17):1994–2001.

4. Katzan IL, Furlan AJ, Lloyd LE, et al. Use of tissue-type plasminogen activator for acute ischemic stroke: the Cleveland area experience. *JAMA*. 2000;283(9): 1151–1158.
5. Lees KR, Bluhmki E, von Kummer R, et al. Time to treatment with intravenous alteplase and outcome in stroke: an updated pooled analysis of ECASS, ATLANTIS, NINDS, and EPITHET trials. *Lancet*. 2010;375(9727):1695–1703.
6. Marler JR, Tilley BC, Lu M, et al. Early stroke treatment associated with better outcome: the NINDS rt-PA stroke study. *Neurology*. 2000;55(11):1649–1655.
7. Physicians ACoE, Neurology AAo. Clinical Policy: Use of intravenous tPA for the management of acute ischemic stroke in the emergency department. *Ann Emerg Med*. 2013;61(2):225–243.

IV Thrombolysis 3 to 4.5 Hours after an Acute Ischemic Stroke

The ECASS III Trial

MICHAEL E. HOCHMAN

> ... [A]lteplase given 3 to 4.5 hours after the onset of stroke symptoms was associated with a modest but significant improvement in the clinical outcome ...
>
> —HACKE ET AL.[1]

Research Question: It has been established that thrombolysis with intravenous alteplase is effective when given within 3 hours of the onset of an acute ischemic stroke; however, is alteplase effective when given 3–4.5 hours after the onset of a stroke?[1]

Funding: The Boehringer Ingelheim Pharmaceutical Company.

Year Study Began: 2003

Year Study Published: 2008

Study Location: More than 100 sites in Europe.

Who Was Studied: Patients 18–80 years old with an acute ischemic stroke presenting within 3 to 4.5 hours after the onset of symptoms.

Who Was Excluded: Patients with evidence of an intracranial hemorrhage on CT or MRI of the brain, those for whom the timing of symptom onset was unknown, those with major surgery or trauma within the previous 3 months, those with a systolic blood pressure >185 mm Hg or a diastolic pressure >110 mm Hg, and those on anticoagulants. Patients with a history of both prior stroke and diabetes were excluded as well. In addition, patients with a "severe stroke," defined as a score >25 on the National Institutes of Health Stroke Scale (NIHSS)[2] or "a stroke involving more than one third of the middle cerebral-artery territory" were excluded, since strokes of this size were considered potentially at higher risk for hemorrhagic transformation.

How Many Patients: 821

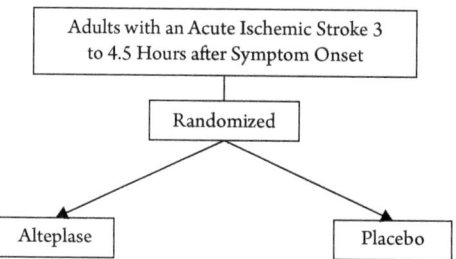

Figure 35.1 Summary of ECASS III's Design.

Study Overview: See Figure 35.1 for a summary of the study design.

Study Intervention: Patients in the alteplase group received 0.9 mg per kg (max dose 90 mg) of alteplase intravenously. Patients in the placebo group received an intravenous placebo. Treatment with intravenous heparin, oral anticoagulants, and aspirin within 24 hours of administration of the study drug was prohibited; however, prophylactic doses of heparin or low-molecular-weight heparin were permitted.

Follow-Up: 90 days.

Endpoints: Primary outcome: disability as assessed using the modified Rankin scale (mRS)[3] (see Table 35.1). Secondary outcomes: disability as assessed using a global disability scale consisting of scores on 4 individual disability scales (mRS, Barthel Index, NIHSS, and Glasgow Outcome Scale); intracranial hemorrhage; and mortality.

Table 35.1. MODIFIED RANKIN SCALE

Score	Description
0	No symptoms
1	Able to carry out all usual activities
2	"Unable to carry out all previous activities, but able to look after own affairs without assistance"
3	"Requiring some help but able to walk without assistance"
4	"Unable to walk without assistance and unable to attend to own bodily needs without assistance"
5	"Bedridden, incontinent and requiring constant nursing care and attention"
6	Dead

Adapted from: http://www.strokecenter.org/trials/scales/rankin.html

RESULTS

- The median time for administration of the study medication following the onset of stroke symptoms was 3 hours and 59 minutes.
- The odds ratio for a positive outcome for alteplase on the global disability scale was 1.28 (95% CI, 1.00–1.65) (see Table 35.2).

Table 35.2. SUMMARY OF ECASS III'S KEY FINDINGS

Outcome	Alteplase Group	Placebo Group	P Value
Favorable outcome on Rankin scale (score 0 or 1)	52.4%	45.2%	0.04
Mortality	7.7%	8.4%	0.68
Intracranial hemorrhage	27.0%	17.6%	0.001
Symptomatic intracranial hemorrhage	2.4%	0.2%	0.008

Criticisms and Limitations:

- Many emergency rooms, including those involved in this trial, have the capability of rapidly determining which patients are appropriate candidates for thrombolysis and administering the therapy quickly. In "real world" settings, however, providing timely thrombolysis for patients presenting with acute strokes remains challenging. It should be noted that the average NIHSS score was lower for patients in this trial than in previous studies, including the NINDS trial[4], a fact that may have helped to select for a population perhaps less likely to have the complication of intracerebral hemorrhage. The other comorbidities excluded, such as age >80 years and prior stroke with diabetes, possibly further helped to reduce the potential complication rate.

Other Relevant Studies and Information:

- The NINDS trial established the benefit of alteplase for acute ischemic strokes within 3 hours of symptom onset.[4] Other trials have failed to show a benefit of thrombolysis up to 6 hours after symptom onset, however.[5-7]
- Despite the fact that thrombolysis appears to be effective up to 4.5 hours after the onset of stroke symptoms, patients treated within the first 1.5 hours appear to have the best outcomes.[8]

Summary and Implications: The ECASS III trial established that thrombolysis with alteplase given up to 4.5 hours after the onset of stroke symptoms is modestly efficacious; however, patients treated within the first 1.5 hours have the best outcomes.

CLINICAL CASE: THROMBOLYSIS FOR ACUTE ISCHEMIC STROKE

Case History:
A 60-year-old woman is rushed to the emergency room by ambulance after her daughter found her at home with slurred speech and weakness of her right arm. The woman called her daughter approximately 2.5 hours prior to arrival in the emergency room because she didn't feel right, but she believes the symptoms actually began 1 hour before calling her daughter.

On examination, the patient's vital signs are unremarkable. She has slurred speech and weakness of the right upper extremity. A CT scan shows possible early ischemic changes involving the left insular cortex, but no hemorrhage. At this point, the patient is now 4 hours after symptom onset. Based on the results of ECASS III, should you treat this patient with thrombolytics?

Suggested Answer:
ECASS III trial established that thrombolysis with alteplase given up to 4.5 hours after the onset of stroke symptoms is modestly efficacious. The patient is currently at 4 hours and has a CT scan without hemorrhage or a large volume of stroke that is already visible. Thus, she should receive thrombolytics if they can be administered immediately.

References

1. Hacke W, Kaste M, Blukmki E, et al. Thrombolysis with alteplase 3 to 4.5 hours after acute ischemic stroke. *N Engl J Med.* 2008;359(13):1317–1329.
2. More information available at: http://www.strokecenter.org/trials/scales/nihss.html.
3. Bonita R, Beaglehole R. Modification of Rankin Scale: Recovery of motor function after stroke. *Stroke.* 1988;19(12):1497–1500.
4. The National Institute of Neurological Disorders and Stroke rt-PA Stroke Study Group. Tissue plasminogen activator for acute ischemic stroke. *N Engl J Med.* 1995;333(24):1581–1587.
5. Hacke W, Kaste M, Fieschi C, et al. Intravenous thrombolysis with recombinant tissue plasminogen activator for acute hemispheric stroke: the European Cooperative Acute Stroke Study (ECASS). *JAMA.* 1995;274:1017-1025.
6. Hacke W, Kaste M, Fieschi C, et al. Randomised double-blind placebo-controlled trial of thrombolytic therapy with intravenous alteplase in acute ischaemic stroke (ECASS II): Second European-Australian Acute Stroke Study Investigators. *Lancet.* 1998;352:1245-1251.
7. Clark WM, Wissman S, Albers GW, et al. Recombinant tissue-type plasminogen activator (alteplase) for ischemic stroke 3 to 5 hours after symptom onset: the ATLANTIS Study: a randomized controlled trial: Alteplase Thrombolysis for Acute Noninterventional Therapy in Ischemic Stroke. *JAMA.* 1999;282:2019-2026.
8. Hacke W, Donnan G, Fieschi C, et al. Association of outcome with early stroke treatment: pooled analysis of ATLANTIS, ECASS, and NINDS rt-PA stroke trials. *Lancet.* 2004;363:768–774.

Endovascular Therapy for Acute Ischemic Stroke, Part I (Intra-arterial Thrombolysis)

The PROACT II Trial

ALLISON ARCH AND DAVID Y. HWANG

> ... treatment with IA r-proUK within 6 hours of the onset of acute ischemic stroke caused by MCA occlusion significantly improved clinical outcomes at 90 days.
> —The PROACT Investigators[1]

Research Question: Is intra-arterial (IA) recombinant prourokinase (r-proUK) plus intravenous heparin effective and safe in patients with acute stroke caused by middle cerebral artery (MCA) occlusion, compared to IV heparin alone?[1]

Funding: Abbott Laboratories.

Year Study Began: 1996

Year Published: 1999

Study Location: 54 centers in North America.

Who Was Studied: Patients aged 18–85 years who had focal neurological signs in the middle cerebral artery (MCA) distribution, could get treatment within

6 hours of stroke symptom onset, and had a minimum National Institutes of Health Stroke Scale (NIHSS) score of 4. Diagnostic cerebral angiography had to show a clot in the M1 or M2 division of the MCA that afforded safe passage of a microcatheter into the MCA.

Who Was Excluded: Patients with an NIHSS >30; rapidly improving neurological signs; recent stroke, surgery, or hemorrhage; current hemorrhage or brain tumor on head computed tomographic (CT) scan; baseline INR >1.7 or activated PTT >1.5 times normal; blood pressure >180/100; patients who could not undergo angiography with contrast.

How Many Patients: 180 patients (121 to the intervention group, and 59 to the control group).

Study Overview: See Figure 36.1 for a summary of the study design.

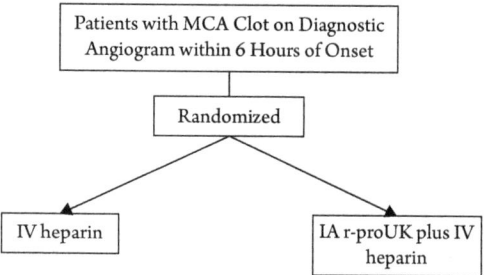

Figure 36.1 Summary of PROACT II's Study Design.

Study Intervention: All enrolled stroke patients who could receive intervention within 6 hours of symptom onset underwent diagnostic angiography. Those who had a visualized clot in the M1 or M2 portion of the MCA were randomized to receive 9 mg of IA r-proUK (as two sequential doses of 4.5 mg) plus IV heparin or IV heparin alone.

Follow-Up: 90 days.

Endpoints: Primary outcome: percentage of patients achieving a modified Rankin score (mRS) of ≤2 at 90 days following therapy. Secondary outcomes: percentage of patients reaching an NIHSS of ≤1 at 90 days, the rates of partial and complete angiographic recanalization defined as TIMI grade 2 or 3 (see Table 36.1), percentage of patients achieving a 50% reduction from baseline NIHSS score at 90 days, hemorrhagic transformation causing neurological deterioration within 24 hours of treatment, procedural complications, and mortality.

Table 36.1. TIMI GRADE FLOW (THROMBOLYSIS IN MYOCARDIAL INFARCTION): A SCORING SYSTEM OF PERFUSION[A]

TIMI Grade	Explanation
0	No perfusion: the absence of any antegrade flow beyond the occlusion
1	Penetration without perfusion: a faint antegrade flow beyond the occlusion, with incomplete filling of the distal bed
2	Partial reperfusion: delayed or sluggish antegrade flow with complete filling of the distal territory
3	Normal flow: the distal bed fills completely

[A] Originally based on the levels of coronary blood flow assessed during percutaneous coronary angioplasty.

RESULTS

- Recanalization rates (TIMI 2 or 3) were 66% for the r-proUK group and 18% for the controls (see Table 36.2).
- Intracranial hemorrhage with neurological deterioration within 24 hours occurred in 10% of the r-proUK patients and 2% of control patients.
- Worsening of neurologic symptoms occurred in 1% of r-proUK cases versus 0% of controls.

Table 36.2. SUMMARY OF PROACT II'S KEY FINDINGS

Outcome (90 day follow-up)	r-proUK group (n = 121; %)	Control (n = 59; %)	Absolute Difference (%)	P value
mRS ≤2	40	25	15	0.04
NIHSS ≥50% decrease	50	44	6	0.46
NIHSS ≤1	18	12	6	0.30
Mortality	25	27	−2	0.80

Criticisms and Limitations: The authors compared IA thrombolysis plus IV heparin to IV heparin alone. However, the standard of care for acute ischemic stroke is not IV heparin. Only 1 patient was treated <3 hours from stroke symptom onset, highlighting practical time challenges with IA therapy at the time this study was conducted. There was also a 2-hour infusion time with r-proUK.

The second 4.5 mg dose of r-proUK was always administered, regardless of whether there was recanalization after administration of the first dose. There was a higher rate of intracranial hemorrhage (10.2%) in PROACT II compared with IV thrombolysis in other multicenter randomized trials. There was also a greater baseline stroke severity (median NIHSS of 17 in PROACT II vs. 14 in the NINDS trial).[2]

Other Relevant Studies and Information:

- While IA r-proUK is not the preferred or currently available option for most interventional neuroradiologists in acute stroke treatment, PROACT II is a historically significant study because it was the first multicenter randomized controlled trial of IA therapy for acute stroke. In the years following PROACT II, several reports described the recanalization rates of newer-generation mechanical thrombectomy devices.[3-5] However, PROACT II remained the only major stroke interventional trial with both a true control arm and clinical outcome data from 1999 until 2013.
- Of note, the success of the PROACT II trial was not enough to gain FDA approval for IA r-proUK, given the high rate of symptomatic intracranial hemorrhage.
- Subsequent clinical trials have looked at the efficacy and safety of intravenous followed by IA thrombolysis for acute stroke. Results have generally shown the feasibility of combination therapy, in addition to improved revascularization rates. Improvements in overall clinical outcome were more variable.[6-9]
- It is worth emphasizing again that current standard of care for acute ischemic stroke is to use intravenous recombinant tissue plasminogen activator for patients who are eligible. Heparin and other anticoagulants are not standard of care treatments in acute stroke, neither in IV nor IA form.[10]

Summary and Implications: PROACT II was the first randomized trial to demonstrate clinical efficacy of IA thrombolysis in patients with acute stroke of <6 hours' duration caused by MCA occlusion, paving the way for a generation of ischemic stroke studies examining the efficacy of various IA treatment approaches and expanding the acute treatment window. One unanticipated result of PROACT II was an ACGME-approved pathway for training interventional neurologists. At the time of publication, PROACT II expanded the stroke treatment window and led directly to the development of mechanical thrombectomy devices, which have now replaced the use of intra-arterial thrombolytics alone. In fact, the first FDA-approved stroke thrombectomy device (MERCI retriever) used the PROACT II data as a historical control.

> **CLINICAL CASE: ENDOVASCULAR THERAPY FOR ACUTE ISCHEMIC STROKE**
>
> Please refer to the case at the end of Chapter 39.

References

1. Furlan A, Higashida R, Wechsler L, et al. Intra-arterial prourokinase for acute ischemic stroke. The PROACT II study: a randomized controlled trial. Prolyse in Acute Cerebral Thromboembolism. *JAMA*. 1999;282(21):2003–2011.
2. Tissue plasminogen activator for acute ischemic stroke. The National Institute of Neurological Disorders and Stroke rt-PA Stroke Study Group. *N Engl J Med*. 1995;333(24):1581–1587.
3. Smith WS, Sung G, Starkman S, et al. Safety and efficacy of mechanical embolectomy in acute ischemic stroke: results of the MERCI trial. *Stroke*. 2005;36(7):1432–1438.
4. Investigators PPST. The penumbra pivotal stroke trial: safety and effectiveness of a new generation of mechanical devices for clot removal in intracranial large vessel occlusive disease. *Stroke*. 2009;40(8):2761–2768.
5. Smith WS, Sung G, Saver J, et al. Mechanical thrombectomy for acute ischemic stroke: final results of the Multi MERCI trial. *Stroke*. 2008;39(4):1205–1212.
6. Lewandowski CA, Frankel M, Tomsick TA, et al. Combined intravenous and intra-arterial r-TPA versus intra-arterial therapy of acute ischemic stroke: Emergency Management of Stroke (EMS) Bridging Trial. *Stroke*. 1999;30(12):2598–2605.
7. Investigators IS. Combined intravenous and intra-arterial recanalization for acute ischemic stroke: the Interventional Management of Stroke Study. *Stroke*. 2004;35(4):904–911.
8. Wolfe T, Suarez JI, Tarr RW, et al. Comparison of combined venous and arterial thrombolysis with primary arterial therapy using recombinant tissue plasminogen activator in acute ischemic stroke. *J Stroke Cerebrovasc Dis*. 2008;17(3):121–128.
9. Flaherty ML, Woo D, Kissela B, et al. Combined IV and intra-arterial thrombolysis for acute ischemic stroke. *Neurology*. 2005;64(2):386–388.
10. Jauch EC, Saver JL, Adams HP, et al. Guidelines for the early management of patients with acute ischemic stroke: a guideline for healthcare professionals from the American Heart Association/American Stroke Association. *Stroke*. 2013;44(3):870–947.

Endovascular Therapy for Acute Ischemic Stroke, Part II (After IV Thrombolysis)

The IMS III Trial

MATTHEW D. KALP AND DAVID Y. HWANG

> The IMS III trial provides preliminary data for a randomized trial to determine whether newer endovascular devices add benefit to intravenous thrombolysis if both therapies can be initiated very early after stroke onset....
> —MARC CHIMOWITZ (ACCOMPANYING EDITORIAL)[1]

Research Question: Should patients that receive intravenous (IV) t-PA for acute ischemic stroke also receive additional endovascular therapy?[2]

Funding: NIH, National Institute of Neurological Disorders and Stroke; also Genentech, EKOS, Concentric Medical, Cordis Neurovascular, and Boehringer Ingelheim.

Year Study Began: 2006

Year Study Published: 2013

Study Location: 58 study centers in the United States, Canada, Australia, and Europe.

Who Was Studied: Patients aged 18–82 years with an acute ischemic stroke that received intravenous t-PA within 3 hours of symptom onset and had an NIHSS score ≥10, or an NIHSS score 8–9 with an occlusion seen in the first segment of the middle cerebral artery (M1), internal carotid artery, or basilar artery on CT angiography (CTA).

Who Was Excluded: Acute stroke patients who did not receive IV t-PA were excluded. Other notable exclusion criteria included seizure at stroke onset, ongoing hemodialysis, and blood glucose level >400 mg/dl. With regard to imaging, patients with a large-territory stroke visible on CT were excluded. Importantly, absence of a major artery occlusion on CTA was only used in the fifth and final protocol of the trial.

How Many Patients: 656 patients.

Study Overview: See Figure 37.1 for a summary of the study design.

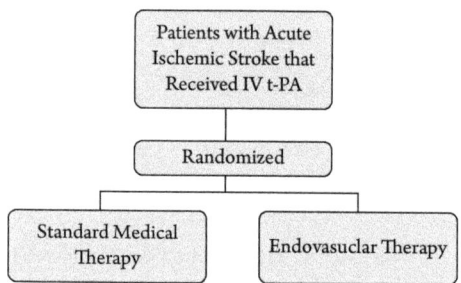

Figure 37.1 Summary of IMS III's Design.

Study Intervention: All patients received IV t-PA for acute ischemic stroke. Within 40 minutes after the initiation of the t-PA infusion, patients were randomly assigned to receive either IV t-PA alone or IV t-PA plus endovascular therapy. Those in the endovascular arm had the IV t-PA infusion stopped at 40 minutes, except for the fifth study protocol in which they received the entire 60 minutes of t-PA infusion. By this point in the trial, safety data about the use of full-dose IV t-PA followed by endovascular therapy had become available. Patients in the combined therapy group underwent catheter angiography, and those with a treatable occlusion received endovascular intervention. Endovascular options, selected by the site neurointerventionalist, included thrombectomy (MERCI retriever, Penumbra System, or Solitaire FR revascularization device) or endovascular delivery of t-PA (Micro-Sonic SV infusion system or a standard catheter). All procedures had to start within 5 hours of stroke ictus and had to finish within 7 hours.

Follow-Up: 90 days.

Endpoints: Primary outcomes: Modified Rankin scale score (mRS) of ≤2. Secondary outcomes included reperfusion rates as measured by the Thrombolysis in Cerebral Infarction (TICI) score (ranges 0–3, with 3 = full reperfusion of the occluded artery), death, intracerebral hemorrhage, major complication due to non-intracerebral bleeding, recurrent stroke, and device or procedural complications.

RESULTS

- This trial was stopped early because of futility. The proportion of patients with an mRS score of ≤2 did not differ significantly between the treatment groups: 40.8% with endovascular therapy and 38.7% with intravenous t-PA. The adjusted absolute difference between the groups was 1.5% with a 95% confidence interval of −6.1 to 9.1. (See Table 37.1.)
- Similarly, there was no statistically significant difference in the treatment groups across the entire mRS distribution for the predefined subgroups of patients with an NIHSS score of ≥20 and those with an NIHSS score of ≤19, although the distribution for the severe stroke subgroup was nearly significant in favor of endovascular therapy ($P = 0.06$).
- Importantly, the overall number of patients in the endovascular arm who achieved a TICI score of 2b or 3 (i.e., at least partial recanalization of half of the occluded artery) was only 44% for M1 occlusions and 38% for terminal ICA occlusions.

Table 37.1. SUMMARY OF IMS III's SAFETY ENDPOINTS

Outcomes	Endovascular Therapy after t-PA	t-PA Alone	P Value
Death within 7 days	12%	10.8%	0.57
Death within 30 days	19.1%	21.6%	0.52
Symptomatic intracerebral hemorrhage	6.2%	5.9%	0.83
Asymptomatic intracerebral hemorrhage	27.4%	18.9%	0.01
Subarachnoid hemorrhage	11.5%	5.8%	0.02
Intraventricular hemorrhage	6.5%	4.8%	0.40
Major complications	3.0%	2.3%	0.55
Recurrent stroke	5.1%	6.3%	0.54

Criticisms and Limitations: IMS III took 5 years to complete prior to study termination because many experts in the stroke community did not feel comfortable randomizing qualified patients to not receive endovascular treatment. This fact may have contributed to a selection bias, removing favorable endovascular candidates from the study.

Only 47% of subjects in IMS III underwent CTA prior to treatment with t-PA. A significant proportion of patients with NIHSS 10–19 may not have had an arterial occlusion amenable to endovascular therapy after receiving IV t-PA. One hundred patients randomized to endovascular treatment (24%) in IMS III did not actually receive endovascular treatment after IV t-PA due to various reasons (e.g., early clinical improvement or deterioration, absence of clot during angiography, and technical failures).

Fourteen percent of the patients in the endovascular group had an ASPECTS (Alberta Stroke Program Early CT Score) of ≤4 on their initial CT, implying that they may have already had an irreversible large territory infarct.[3] ASPECTS is a 10-point scale used to judge the extent of ischemic stroke in the MCA territory on a noncontrast CT, with 10 being a normal CT and 0 representing early ischemic changes in the entire MCA territory.

Because IMS III took several years to enroll and the technology was rapidly changing, the devices used for endovascular therapy were no longer "cutting edge" by its completion. Only a few patients were treated with newer stent retriever devices when it became an FDA-cleared and study-approved device just prior to stopping the study for futility. Older devices, such as the MERCI retriever, or intra-arterial t-PA were used in most patients.

Other Relevant Studies and Information:

- An editorial accompanying the publication of IMS III pointed out that the subgroup of endovascular patients who received IV tPA within 2 hours of stroke symptoms and underwent the procedure within 90 minutes of tPA had a possible, but not statistically significant, outcome benefit.[1]
- Predefined 12-month outcome data for IMS III demonstrated a significant benefit for subjects with an NIHSS score > 19 in favor of endovascular therapy.[4]
- In a post-hoc analysis of IMS III patients that underwent CTA prior to treatment with t-PA, there was evidence of a potential benefit for endovascular therapy at 90 days ($P = 0.01$) which was seen most clearly in patients with a terminal ICA occlusion.[5]

Summary and Implications: IMS III failed to show a benefit in 90-day functional outcome of IV t-PA plus endovascular therapy versus IV t-PA alone for acute ischemic stroke. Safety endpoints, notably death and symptomatic intracerebral hemorrhage, were largely similar in both groups. While more recent studies have now shown an outcome benefit for endovascular therapy for certain stroke patients, mostly using stent retrievers and more selective patient enrollment criteria, IMS III remains a landmark trial and a case study in the influence of clinical trial design on study results.

CLINICAL CASE: ENDOVASCULAR THERAPY FOR ACUTE ISCHEMIC STROKE

Please refer to the case at the end of Chapter 39.

References

1. Chimowitz MI. Endovascular treatment for acute ischemic stroke—still unproven. *N Engl J Med.* 2013;368:952–955.
2. Broderick JP, Palesch YY, Demchuk AM, et al. Endovascular therapy after intravenous t-PA versus t-PA alone for stroke. *N Engl J Med.* 2013;368:893–903.
3. Hill MD, Demchuk AM, Goyal M. Alberta Stroke Program early computed tomography score to select patients for endovascular treatment: Interventional Management of Stroke (IMS)-III Trial. *Stroke.* 2014;45:444–449.
4. Palesch YY, Yeatts SD, Tomsick, TA, et al. Twelve-month clinical and quality-of-life outcomes in the Interventional Management of Stroke III Trial. *Stroke.* 2015;46(5):1321–1327. doi:10.1161/STROKEAHA.115009180.
5. Demchuk AM, Goyal M, Yeatts SD, et al. Recanalization and clinical outcome of occlusion sites at baseline CT angiography in the Interventional Management of Stroke III Trial. Radiology 2014;273:202–210.

Endovascular Therapy for Acute Ischemic Stroke, Part III (Using Neuroimaging to Select Patients)

The MR RESCUE Trial

MATTHEW D. KALP AND DAVID Y. HWANG

> Since the MR RESCUE study...[that tested]...the ischemic-penumbra hypothesis...was limited by the small sample size and and use of less effective thrombectomy devices,...[newer] randomized trials will be needed to retest this hypothesis with the use of newer devices once the accuracy of perfusion imaging for identifying viable brain tissue has been more clearly established.
> —MARK CHIMOWITZ (ACCOMPANYING EDITORIAL)[1]

Research Question: Can neuroimaging identify acute stroke patients who are most likely to have improved clinical outcomes from endovascular mechanical embolectomy?[2]

Funding: National Institutes of Neurological Disorders and Stroke.

Year Study Began: 2004

Year Study Published: 2013

Study Location: 22 sites in North America.

Who Was Studied: Patients between age 18–85 years with National Institutes of Health Stroke Scale (NIHSS) scores of 6–29 who presented with large vessel proximal anterior circulation occlusion on MR or CT angiography (distal internal carotid artery, M1 segment of the middle cerebral artery [MCA], or M2 segment of the MCA) within 8 hours of symptom onset.

Who Was Excluded: Patients with a contraindication to MRI (i.e., pacemaker); acute intracranial hemorrhage; coma; rapidly improving neurological signs prior to randomization; preexisting medical, neurological, or psychiatric disease that would confound the neurological, functional, or imaging evaluations; pregnancy; contrast allergy; proximal ICA occlusion; proximal carotid stenosis >67%; dissection; INR > 3.0; PTT > 3 times the normal range; renal failure.

How Many Patients: 118 patients

Study Overview: See Figure 38.1 for a summary of the study design.

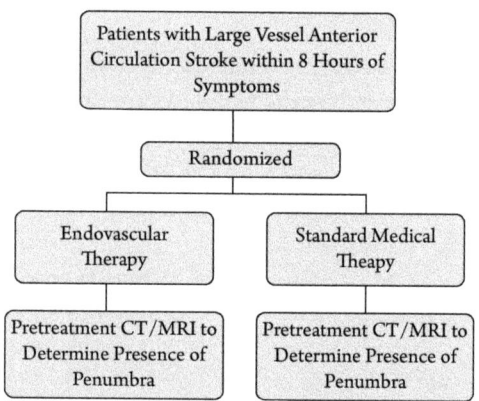

Figure 38.1 Summary of MR RESCUE's Design.

Study Intervention: Regardless of treatment group, all patients underwent a multimodal CT or MRI (i.e., perfusion imaging) of the brain that stratified them based on the presence of a favorable penumbral pattern versus nonpenumbral pattern. An "unfavorable penumbral" pattern was defined as a visible infarct larger than 90 cc or >70% of the presumed perfusion territory at risk. Patients in the mechanical embolectomy arm underwent treatment with either the MERCI Retriever, Penumbra System or both, with intra-arterial t-PA as a second-line treatment. Treatment with IV t-PA did not exclude a patient from undergoing mechanical embolectomy if assigned to that treatment group.

Follow-Up: 90 days.

Outcomes: Primary outcomes: Interaction of the pretreatment penumbral pattern on neuroimaging with all levels of the modified Rankin Scale (mRS) score (0–6), compared between treatment groups. Secondary outcomes: mean and median mRS, mRS scores 0–2, partial revascularization status based on the Thrombolysis in Cerebral Infarction scale (TICI; 2a–3 of a 3-point scale, or at least some partial filling of entire distal vascular bed), day 7 reperfusion (reduction of >90% of the perfusion lesion on MRI), adverse events, and mortality.

RESULTS

- The difference in the 90-day mRS distribution between those patients with a favorable penumbra on neuroimaging versus those with an unfavorable pattern was statistically the same among those patients undergoing endovascular therapy as those receiving standard care (mean difference 0.88, $P = 0.14$).
- Overall, there was no significant outcome difference between patients in the standard care and embolectomy groups (regardless of neuroimaging findings) on the basis of the 90-day mean mRS score (3.9 vs. 3.9, $P = 0.99$) (see Table 38.1).

Table 38.1. SUMMARY OF MR RESCUE's KEY FINDINGS

Outcome	Embolectomy, Penumbral	Standard Care, Penumbral	Embolectomy, Nonpenumbral	Standard Care, Nonpenumbral	P Value
Partial/complete revascularization	67%	93%	77%	78%	0.13
Day 7 reperfusion	57%	52%	37%	50%	0.59
Median final infarct volume (mL)	58.1	37.3	172.6	217.1	<0.001
Mean 90-day mRS	3.9	3.4	4.0	4.4	0.23
mRS[a] 0–2 90 days	21%	26%	17%	10%	0.48
Death	18%	21%	20%	30%	0.75
Symptomatic hemorrhage	9%	6%	0%	0%	0.24

[a] Modified Rankin Scale.

Study Limitations: The trial suffered from a low sample size for its 4-way analysis and a slow recruitment rate: 22 participating centers enrolled 118 patients during the 2004–2011 period, or 1 patient every 8 months. This slow rate was secondary to difficulty with equipoise in randomization among site investigators, in the setting of readily available endovascular devices that had already been granted approval from the FDA.

The definition of "partial" revascularization in this study, a TICI score of 2a–3, was very liberal. A stricter definition of a TICI score of 2b–3, where all of the vascular bed distal to an occlusion is seen to fill (albeit perhaps slowly), would have given this trial a revascularization rate of just 27%. The study used first-generation endovascular devices, which achieve lower rates of recanalization compared to newer stent retrievers.[3,4] A good clinical outcome, defined as a 90-day mRS of ≤2, was only achieved in 19% of the endovascular patients, versus 42% in IMS III. This is partly due to a shorter enrollment window in IMS III and different inclusion/exclusion criteria.

Other Relevant Studies and Information:

- The appropriate infarct size cutoff to define favorable penumbral imaging is debated in the literature. Whereas the infarct "size cutoff" in MR RESCUE was 90 cc, some centers have argued that the size cutoff should be as low as 50 cc.[5]
- Prior to the release of newer randomized trials of endovascular therapy with positive results, the multicenter DEFUSE 2 study looked at clinical outcomes of patients undergoing endovascular therapy with a favorable versus unfavorable penumbral pattern (e.g., restricted diffusion lesion < 70 cc and > 70 cc), with no nonendovascular treatment arm, and found a significant benefit in clinical outcomes for patients with the favorable pattern.[6]

Summary and Implications: The MR RESCUE study attempted to utilize advanced neuroimaging to identify stroke patients most likely to benefit from endovascular therapy. In the context of newer positive trials that do show an outcome benefit for endovascular therapy, MR RESCUE is a case study in how selection bias, thresholds for penumbral definitions, time to treatment, and recanalization rates can effect stroke trial outcome.

CLINICAL CASE: ENDOVASCULAR THERAPY FOR ACUTE ISCHEMIC STROKE

Please refer to the case at the end of Chapter 39.

References

1. Chimowitz MI. Endovascular treatment for acute ischemic stroke—still unproven. *N Engl J Med*. 2013;368:952–955.
2. Kidwell CS, Jahan R, Gornbein J, et al. A trial of imaging selection and endovascular treatment for ischemic stroke. *N Engl J Med*. 2013;368:914–923.
3. Nogueira RG, Lutsep HL, Gupta R, et al. Trevo versus Merci retrievers for thrombectomy revascularisation of large vessel occlusions in acute ischaemic stroke (TREVO 2): a randomised trial. *Lancet*. 2012;380:1231–1240.
4. Saver JL, Jahan R, Levy EI, et al. Solitaire flow restoration device versus the Merci Retriever in patients with acute ischaemic stroke (SWIFT): a randomised, parallel-group, non-inferiority trial. *Lancet*. 2012;380:1241–1249.
5. Yoo AJ, Chaudhry ZA, Nogueira RG, et al. Infarct volume is a pivotal biomarker after intra-arterial stroke therapy. *Stroke*. 2012;43:1323–1330.
6. Lansberg MG, Straka M, Kemp S, et al. MRI profile and response to endovascular reperfusion after stroke (DEFUSE 2): a prospective cohort study. *Lancet Neurol*. 2012;11:860–867.

Endovascular Therapy for Acute Ischemic Stroke, Part IV (Clinical Trial Success)

The MR CLEAN Trial

MATTHEW D. KALP AND DAVID Y. HWANG

In patients with acute ischemic stroke caused by a proximal intracranial occlusion of the anterior circulation, intraarterial treatment administered within 6 hours after stroke onset was effective and safe.
—Berkhemer et al.[1]

Research Question: Do patients with an acute ischemic stroke due to a proximal occlusion of the anterior cerebral circulation benefit from intra-arterial (IA) treatment within 6 hours of symptom onset?[1]

Funding: Dutch Heart Foundation; also the AngioCare Covidien/ev3, Medac/Lamepro, and Penumbra companies.

Year Study Began: 2010

Year Study Published: 2015

Study Location: 16 study centers in the Netherlands.

Who Was Studied: Patients age 18 and older with an acute ischemic stroke (NIHSS ≥ 2) due to a proximal arterial occlusion in the anterior cerebral circulation (i.e., distal internal carotid artery, M1, M2, A1, A2 segments) that was confirmed on vessel imaging and that could undergo IA treatment within 6 hours of symptom onset.

Who Was Excluded: Standard exclusion criteria for IV t-PA were used in addition to specific criteria for mechanical thrombectomy and IA thrombolysis, including history of intracerebral hemorrhage, history of severe head injury within the previous 4 weeks, and clinical or laboratory evidence of coagulation abnormalities.

How Many Patients: 500

Study Overview: See Figure 39.1 for a summary of the study design.

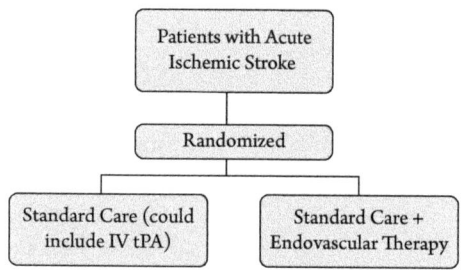

Figure 39.1 Summary of MR CLEAN's Design.

Study Intervention: Patients were randomized to IA treatment (mechanical thrombectomy, IA thrombolysis, or both) plus standard care versus standard care alone. In both arms, "standard care" could include IV tPA. The method of IA treatment was selected by the neurointerventionalist. Alteplase or urokinase were allowed as the IA thrombolytic agent, with maximum doses of 90 mg/30 mg or 1,200,000 IU/400,000 IU (with/without IV t-PA), respectively. Options for mechanical treatment included thrombus retraction, aspiration, wire disruption, or use of a retrievable stent. Initiation of IA therapy had to start within 6 hours of stroke ictus.

Follow-Up: 90 days.

Endpoints: Primary outcome: Shift in the distribution of the modified Rankin Scale (mRS) scores at 90 days. Secondary outcomes included the NIHSS score at 24 hours and at 5 to 7 days (or discharge, if earlier), functional outcome measured with the Barthel index, and health-related quality of life measured with the EuroQol Group 5-Dimension Self-Report Questionnaire at 90 days. Other outcomes assessed included arterial recanalization measured with CTA or MRA at 24 hours, the final infarct volume on noncontrast CT at 5 to 7 days, hemorrhagic complications, progression of ischemic stroke, new ischemic stroke into a different vascular territory, and mortality.

RESULTS

- The median ASPECTS score for enrolled patients was 9, implying that most patients had initial head CTs without large territories of stroke already visible. The ASPECTS score is explained in Chapter 38.
- The majority of patients in the treatment arm underwent thrombectomy via a retrievable stent as first-line therapy.
- When compared to standard care, IA treatment shifted the mRS scores toward better outcomes for all categories except death, with an adjusted common odds ratio of 1.67 (95% confidence interval, 1.21–2.30).
- About 33% of patients who received IA treatment, versus 19% of patients who received standard care, achieved an mRS score between 0 to 2 (see Table 39.1).
- No significant difference was observed between groups with respect to serious adverse events.
- The treatment effect—improvement in the mRS scores—was observed across a variety of subgroups, including those grouped by age, NIHSS score, and ASPECTS score.
- All clinical and imaging outcomes favored IA therapy (see Table 39.2).

Table 39.1. PROPORTION OF PATIENTS IN EACH mRS CATEGORY AT 90 DAYS

mRS Score	Endovascular Intervention (n = 233) (%)	Controls (n = 267) (%)
0 (no deficit)	3	0
1	9	6
2	21	13
3	18	16
4	22	30
5	6	12
6 (death)	21	22

Table 39.2. MR CLEAN'S SECONDARY OUTCOMES

Outcome	Intervention (n = 233)	Control (n = 267)	Effect Variable	Unadjusted Value (95% CI)
NIHSS score after 24 hr	13 (6–20)	16 (12–21)	Beta	2.6 (1.2–4.1)
NIHSS score at 5–7 days or discharge	8 (2–17)	14 (7–18)	Beta	3.2 (1.7–4.7)
Barthel index of 19 or 20 at 90 days	99/215	73/245	Odds ratio	2.0 (1.3–2.9)
EQ-5D score at 90 days	0.69	0.66	Beta	0.08 (0.00–0.15)
No intracranial occlusion on follow-up angiography	141/187	68/207	Odds ratio	6.27 (4.03–9.74)
Final infarct volume (mL)	49	79	Beta	20 (3–36)

Criticisms and Limitations: Whereas 92% of patients in the endovascular treatment group had a complete occlusion at presentation (modified Thrombolysis in Cerebral Infarction [mTICI] score of 0), only 59% had good flow (mTICI score of 2b or 3) after the intervention. In contrast, recent case series of stent retrievers report recanalization rates of 80% or higher.[2,3] Despite the positive results of the trial, IA treatment was not without risk: 5.6% of the patients in the intervention group had embolization into new vascular territories on digital subtraction angiography. There are also concerns about the generalizability of the results. MR CLEAN was conducted at 30 centers within the Netherlands, a small country. This allowed for most patients to access a hospital within a half hour and receive IV tPA. These results might not be easily replicable in countries with wider distances between qualified centers, the population of patients who do not receive IV tPA needs to be further studied.

Other Relevant Studies and Information:

- MR CLEAN was published following the attention garnered by the IMS III, SYNTHESIS Expansion, and MR RESCUE studies, which failed to show the benefit of endovascular procedures over standard intravenous thrombolysis.[4-6] Unlike IMS III and SYNTHESIS Expansion, MR CLEAN required a visualized proximal intracranial occlusion for study eligibility. On average, patients in MR CLEAN had higher ASPECTS scores and faster times to groin puncture. The use of stent retrievers as opposed to the older devices led to higher TICI 2b/3 recanalization rates.

- IMS III and MR RESCUE enrolled 1 or 2 patients per year per center, suggesting that some patients received endovascular therapy outside of the trials, and hence a selection bias.[4,6] However, all of the Dutch centers that provided IA treatment participated in the trial, which was a requirement for reimbursement by insurance companies.[7]
- Four other similar studies (and counting) of endovascular therapy for acute ischemic stroke, ESCAPE,[8] EXTEND-IA,[9] SWIFT-PRIME,[10] and REVASCAT,[11] were stopped early because of efficacy and were published shortly after MR CLEAN. Each of these studies had different time windows for treatment, with ESCAPE enrolling patients up to 12 hours after symptom onset. Of note, for all 4 of these studies, and in contrast to MR CLEAN, strict criteria were reported for selecting patients likely to benefit by radiographic criteria, whether by assessing ASPECTS, CTA collaterals, or burden of stroke and penumbra seen on advanced neuroimaging.

Summary and Implications: MR CLEAN is the first of a number of studies demonstrating that IA treatment within 6 hours of onset of acute ischemic stroke caused by a proximal intracranial occlusion of the anterior circulation improves outcome. There was no difference between treatment and control groups for mortality and symptomatic intracranial hemorrhage.

CLINICAL CASE: ENDOVASCULAR THERAPY FOR ACUTE ISCHEMIC STROKE

Case History:
A 67-year-old woman with a history of hypertension presents to the emergency department 70 minutes after she developed right-sided weakness and word-finding difficulties. Her initial NIHSS score is 15. A noncontrast CT shows an ASPECTS score of 10 (no visible hypodensity). A CT angiogram reveals a left-sided occlusion of the M1 segment of her left middle cerebral artery. How should the acute stroke team manage this patient?

Suggested Answer:
The patient should receive full-dose intravenous t-PA without delay if there are no contraindications. The patient is presenting very early after the onset of symptoms, and has a known M1 occlusion, a high NIHSS score, and a CT scan without evidence of significant ischemia. This patient should proceed to endovascular therapy using a stent-retriever without delay. If the patient were to present further out from her initial onset of symptoms (especially if time to groin puncture would exceed 6 hours from time of stroke onset), and especially if her initial CT or CTA were to suggest a developing infarct or poor collateral circulation, careful thought would need to be paid to her likelihood to benefit from the intervention.

References

1. Berkhemer OA, Fransen PS, Beumer D, et al. A randomized trial of intraarterial treatment for acute ischemic stroke. *N Engl J Med*. 2015;372:11–20.
2. Saver JL, Jahan R, Levy EI, et al. Solitaire flow restoration device versus the Merci Retriever in patients with acute ischaemic stroke (SWIFT): a randomised, parallel-group, non-inferiority trial. *Lancet*. 2012;380:1241–1249.
3. Nogueira RG, Lutsep HL, Gupta R, et al. Trevo versus Merci retrievers for thrombectomy revascularisation of large vessel occlusions in acute ischaemic stroke (TREVO 2): a randomised trial. Lancet 2012;380:1231–1240.
4. Broderick JP, Palesch YY, Demchuk AM, et al. Endovascular therapy after intravenous t-PA versus t-PA alone for stroke. *N Engl J Med*. 2013;368:893–903.
5. Ciccone A, Valvassori L, Nichelatti M, et al. Endovascular treatment for acute ischemic stroke. *N Engl J Med*. 2013;368:904–913.
6. Kidwell CS, Jahan R, Gornbein J, et al. A trial of imaging selection and endovascular treatment for ischemic stroke. *N Engl J Med*. 2013;368:914–923.
7. Hacke W. Interventional thrombectomy for major stroke—a step in the right direction. *N Engl J Med*. 2015;372:76–77.
8. Goyal M, Demchuk AM, Menon BK, et al. Randomized assessment of rapid endovascular treatment of acute stroke. *N Engl J Med*. 2015;372:1019–1030. doi:10.1056/NEJMoa1414905.
9. Campbell BCV, Mitchell PJ, Kleinig TJ, et al. Endovascular therapy for ischemic stroke with perfusion-imaging selection. *N Engl J Med*. 2015;372:1009–1018. doi:10.1056/NEJMoa1414792.
10. Saver JL, Goyal M, Bonafe A, et al. Stent-retriever thrombectomy after intravenous t-PA vs. t-PA alone in stroke. *N Engl J Med*. 2015;372:2295–2295. doi:10.1056/NEJMoa1415061.
11. Jovin TG, Chamorro A, Cobo E, et al. Thrombectomy within 8 hours after symptom onset in ischemic stroke. *N Engl J Med*. 2015;372:2296–2306. doi:10.1056/NEJM1503780.

Carotid Endarterectomy for Symptomatic High-Grade Carotid Stenosis

The NASCET Trial, Part I

HARDIK P. AMIN

> Carotid endarterectomy is highly beneficial to patients with recent hemispheric and retinal transient ischemic attacks or nondisabling strokes and ipsilateral high-grade stenosis (70 to 99 percent) of the internal carotid artery...
>
> —THE NASCET INVESTIGATORS[1]

Research Question: Does carotid endarterectomy reduce the risk of future stroke among patients with a recent adverse cerebrovascular event with ipsilateral high-grade carotid stenosis?[1]

Funding: National Institute of Neurological Disorders and Stroke; aspirin provided by SmithKline Beecham.

Year Study Began: 1987

Year Study Published: 1991

Study Location: 50 clinical centers in the United States and Canada.

Who Was Studied: "Patients who were: (1) less than 80 years of age; (2) had a hemispheric transient attack with distinct focal neurological dysfunction or monocular blindness for < 24 hours; (3) had a non-disabling stroke with persistence of symptoms for > 24 hours within previous 120 days, with 30–99% stenosis of the ipsilateral carotid artery."[1] While the entire NASCET trial was thus designed to enroll a wide range of patients with regard to degree of carotid stenosis, the results for those patients with a stenosis of 70%–99% were published first for reasons outlined below.

Who Was Excluded: "Patients who (1) were mentally incompetent or unwilling to consent; (2) had no angiographic visualization of both carotid arteries and their intracranial branches; (3) had an intracranial lesion that was more severe than the surgically accessible lesion; (4) had organ failure or terminal cancer; (5) had an ischemic stroke that deprived the patient of all useful function in the affected territory; (6) had symptoms that could be attributable to a non-atherosclerotic disease process such as fibromuscular dysplasia, aneurysm or tumor; (7) had a cardiac valvular or rhythm disorder that would raise concern for a cardioembolic process; (8) had already undergone an ipsilateral carotid endarterectomy."[1]

How Many Patients: 659

Study Overview: See Figure 40.1 for a summary of the study design.

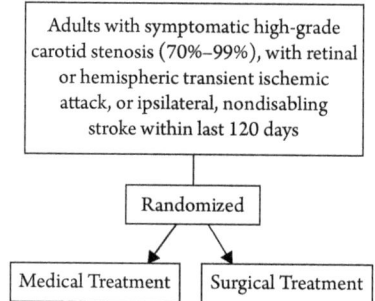

Figure 40.1 Summary of NASCET's (Part I) Design.

Study Intervention: Patients randomized to the medical treatment group received antiplatelet therapy (usually aspirin), and, if indicated, antihypertensive and antilipidemic drugs. Patients randomized to the surgical group underwent carotid endarterectomy of the stenotic vessel, with surgical technique left to the discretion of the individual surgeon.

Follow-Up: Postoperative assessments were performed by study surgeons 30 days after surgery or at hospital discharge (whichever occurred first). Medical, neurological, and functional status assessments were performed by study neurologists 1 month after trial entry, then every 3 months for the first year, and every 4 months thereafter. The average duration of follow-up for patients with high-grade stenosis (70%–99%) was 18 months.

Endpoints: Primary endpoint: any stroke or death in the perioperative period, plus ipsilateral stroke beyond the perioperative period.

RESULTS

- The original trial's preplanned rule for stopping randomization was invoked because of evidence of treatment efficacy among patients with high-grade stenosis (70%–99%) who underwent carotid endarterectomy. Thus, enrollment for high-grade stenosis ended in 1991, while patients with moderate stenosis continued to be enrolled (see Chapter 41).
- For patients with high-grade stenosis, surgically treated patients had a 2.1% risk of major stroke and death in the perioperative period (time from randomization to 30 days after surgery).
- Medically treated patients had a 0.9% risk of major stroke in a comparable 32-day period after randomization.
- Surgically treated patients had a 9% risk of *any* fatal or nonfatal ipsilateral stroke by 24 months after randomization and a 2.5% risk of major or fatal stroke. Medically treated patients had a 26% risk of *any* fatal or nonfatal ipsilateral stroke by 24 months after randomization and a 13% risk of major or fatal stroke. Carotid endarterectomy was associated with an absolute risk reduction of:
  - 17% for cumulative risk of any ipsilateral stroke at 2 years (±3.5%, $P < 0.001$)
  - 10.6% for cumulative risk of major or fatal ipsilateral stroke at 2 years (±2.6%, $P < 0.001$)

Criticisms and Limitations: Criticisms of this trial include the exclusion of many high-risk patients (such as >80 years old in the high-grade stenosis arm), the use of highly selected surgeons, and the lack of independent neurological evaluations.[2] This trial was also conducted in an era where statin use was not as widespread. Many advocate repeating the study using modern standards of best medical therapy.

Other Relevant Studies and Information:

- The European Carotid Surgery Trial (ECST) was a randomized controlled trial that allocated 3,024 patients with some degree of carotid stenosis and recent ipsilateral ischemic vascular event to surgery or conservative management. The trial demonstrated a benefit of surgery among patients with a carotid stenosis >80%; however, methods of calculating stenosis differed between the two trials.[3]

Summary and Implications: NASCET was the first large North American randomized controlled trial to provide evidence demonstrating the benefits of carotid endarterectomy for patients with high-grade carotid stenosis (70%–99%). There was, however, substantial perioperative risk among this patient population.

- Based on the results of this trial and the European Carotid Surgery trial, guidelines from the American Heart Association/American Stroke Association recommend that "for patients with a TIA or ischemic stroke within the past 6 months and ipsilateral severe (70%–99%) carotid artery stenosis as documented by noninvasive imaging, CEA is recommended if the perioperative morbidity and mortality risk is estimated to be <6%."[4]

CLINICAL CASE: CAROTID ENDARTERECTOMY FOR SYMPTOMATIC CAROTID STENOSIS

Please refer to the case at the end of Chapter 41 ("The NASCET Trial, Part II").

References

1. Collaborators NASCET. Beneficial effect of carotid endarterectomy in symptomatic patients with high-grade carotid stenosis. *N Engl J Med.* 1991;325:445–453.
2. Hallett JW, Pietropaoli JA, Ilstrup DM, Gayari MM, Williams JA, Meyer FB. Comparison of North American Symptomatic Carotid Endarterectomy Trial and population-based outcomes for carotid endarterectomy. *J Vasc Surg.* 1998;27: 845–850; discussion 851.

3. Randomised trial of endarterectomy for recently symptomatic carotid stenosis: final results of the MRC European Carotid Surgery Trial (ECST). *Lancet.* 1998;351:1379–1387.
4. Kernan W, Obviagele B, Black HR, et al. Guidelines for the prevention of stroke in patients with stroke and transient ischemic attack: a guideline for healthcare professionals from the American Heart Association/American Stroke Association. *Stroke* 2014;45(7):2160–2236.

41

Carotid Endarterectomy for Symptomatic Moderate Carotid Stenosis

The NASCET Trial, Part II

HARDIK P. AMIN

> Endarterectomy in patients with symptomatic moderate carotid stenosis of 50 to 69 percent yielded only a moderate reduction in the risk of stroke...
>
> —THE NASCET INVESTIGATORS[1]

Research Question: Does carotid endarterectomy reduce the risk of future stroke or death in patients with symptomatic moderate carotid stenosis, defined as less than 70%?[1]

Funding: National Institute of Neurological Disorders and Stroke; aspirin provided by SmithKline Beecham.

Year Study Began: 1987

Year Study Published: 1998

Study Location: 50 clinical centers in the United States and Canada.

Who Was Studied: "Patients who had (1) focal cerebral ischemia ipsilateral to a stenosis of less than 70% in the internal carotid artery within 180 days, as shown on selective angiograph; (2) persisting less than 24 hours or producing a non-disabling stroke."[1]

Who Was Excluded: "Patients who (1) were mentally incompetent or unwilling to consent; (2) lacked angiographic visualization of the symptomatic artery; (3) had an intracranial lesion that was more severe than the surgically accessible lesion; (4) other disease that limited life expectancy to less than five years; (5) had cerebral infarction that eliminated useful function in the affected territory; (6) non-atherosclerotic disease process such as fibromuscular dysplasia, aneurysm or tumor; (7) had a cardiac valvular or rhythm disorder that would raise concern for a cardio-embolic process; (8) had already undergone an ipsilateral carotid endarterectomy."[1]

How Many Patients: 2,226

Study Overview: See Figure 41.1 for a summary of the study design.

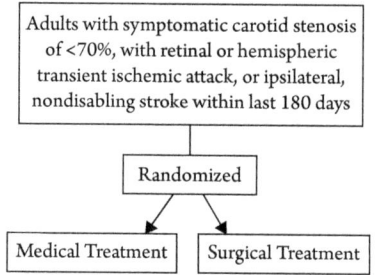

Figure 41.1 Summary of NASCET's Design.

Study Intervention: Patients randomized to the medical treatment group received antiplatelet therapy (usually aspirin), and if indicated, antihypertensive and antilipidemic drugs. Patients randomized to the surgical group underwent carotid endarterectomy of the stenotic vessel, with surgical technique left to the discretion of the individual surgeon.

Follow-Up: Postoperative assessments were performed by study surgeons 30 days after surgery or at hospital discharge (whichever occurred first). Medical, neurological, and functional status assessments were performed by study neurologists 1 month after trial entry, then every 3 months for the first year, and every 4 months thereafter. The mean follow-up for patients with moderate stenosis (<70%) was 5 years.

Endpoints: Primary endpoint: any stroke or death in the perioperative period, plus ipsilateral stroke beyond the perioperative period.

RESULTS

Primary and Secondary Outcomes for Patients with Moderate (≤70%) Stenosis:

- Among patients with 50%–69% stenosis, the 5-year ipsilateral stroke risk was moderately lower among patients treated surgically than those treated with medical therapy alone (see Table 41.1).
- Patients with stenosis <50% did not benefit from surgery. (see Table 41.1)
- The overall rate of perioperative stroke and death was 6.5% in the surgical therapy group. The rate of permanently disabling stroke and death was 2.0%.[1]
- The most common surgical complication was cranial nerve injury, followed by wound hematoma.
- The upper age limit of 80 was removed for this section of the trial.
- Surgical intervention afforded patients with 50%–69% stenosis a 29% relative risk reduction (95% confidence interval, 7%–52%).

Table 41.1. ANY IPSILATERAL STROKE AT 5 YEARS (%)

Stenosis	Surgical Group	Medical Group	P value
50%–69%	15.7%	22.2%	0.045
<50%	14.9%	18.7%	0.16

Criticisms and Limitations: Criticisms of this trial include the exclusion of many high-risk patients (e.g., ≥80 years old in the high-grade stenosis arm), the use of highly selected surgeons, and the lack of independent neurological evaluations.[2] This trial was also conducted in an era where statin use was not as widespread. Many advocate repeating the study using modern standards of best medical therapy.

Other Relevant Studies and Information:

- The European Carotid Surgery Trial (ECST) was a randomized controlled trial that allocated 3,024 patients with some degree of carotid stenosis and recent ipsilateral ischemic vascular event to surgery or conservative management. The trial demonstrated a benefit of surgery among patients with a carotid stenosis >80%; however, methods of calculating stenosis differed between the two trials.[3]

Summary and Implications: NASCET was the first large North American randomized controlled trial to provide evidence demonstrating a benefit of surgery among patients with moderate stenosis (50%–69%). There was substantial perioperative risk among this patient population, however.

- Based on the results of this trial and the European Carotid Surgery Trial, guidelines from the American Heart Association/American Stroke Association recommend that "for patients with recent TIA or ischemic stroke and ipsilateral moderate (50%–69%) carotid stenosis as documented by catheter-based imaging or noninvasive imaging with corroboration (eg, magnetic resonance angiogram or computed tomography angiogram), [carotid endarterectomy] is recommended depending on patient-specific factors, such as age, sex, and comorbidities, if the perioperative morbidity and mortality risk is estimated to be <6%" (class I; level of evidence B).[4]

CLINICAL CASE: CAROTID ENDARTERECTOMY FOR SYMPTOMATIC CAROTID STENOSIS

Case History:
A 70-year-old man with a history of hypercholesterolemia, hypertension, smoking, and obesity presents with a recent episode of right-sided arm and leg weakness and expressive speech difficulties. This occurred about 3 weeks ago, and the episode lasted 10–15 minutes in total, after which his symptoms completely resolved. He did not seek medical attention immediately, but saw his primary doctor 1 week later. He tells you that a similar event may have happened last year, but perhaps not as severe. A carotid Doppler revealed <50% stenosis in his right internal carotid artery, and at least 70% stenosis in the left internal carotid artery. CT scan of the brain demonstrated significant periventricular small vessel disease, and subacute bilateral lacunar infarcts. He has been taking aspirin 81 mg daily for the past 10 years.

Based on the trial results, what would you recommend to this patient?

Suggested Answer:
This patient has many cardiovascular risk factors, including hyperlipidemia, hypertension, obesity, and a history of smoking. He already has evidence of chronic ischemia on his CT scan in the form of small vessel disease and lacunar infarcts, and therefore needs to be counseled on multiple lifestyle modifications. His recent syndrome of aphasia with weakness localizes to the left middle cerebral artery territory, likely as a result of his proximal internal carotid artery stenosis. Based on NASCET results, a left carotid endarterectomy should be considered for this patient. Given the perioperative risks, this decision should be shared between the patient and his physician.

References

1. Barnett HJ, Taylor DW, Eliasziw M, et al. Benefit of carotid endarterectomy in patients with symptomatic moderate or severe stenosis. North American Symptomatic Carotid Endarterectomy Trial Collaborators. *N Engl J Med.* 1998;339:1415–1425.
2. Hallett JW, Pietropaoli JA, Ilstrup DM, Gayari MM, Williams JA, Meyer FB. Comparison of North American Symptomatic Carotid Endarterectomy Trial and population-based outcomes for carotid endarterectomy. *J Vasc Surg.* 1998;27:845–850; discussion 851.
3. Randomised trial of endarterectomy for recently symptomatic carotid stenosis: final results of the MRC European Carotid Surgery Trial (ECST). *Lancet.* 1998;351:1379–1387.
4. Kernan W, Obviagele B, Black HR, et al. Guidelines for the prevention of stroke in patients with stroke and transient ischemic attack: a guideline for healthcare professionals from the American Heart Association/American Stroke Association. *Stroke* 2014;45(7):2160–2236.

Carotid Endarterectomy for Asymptomatic Carotid Stenosis
The ACAS Trial

DANIEL C. BROOKS

> Patients with asymptomatic carotid artery stenosis of 60% or greater reduction in diameter . . . will have a reduced 5-year risk of ipsilateral stroke if carotid endarterectomy performed with less than 3% perioperative morbidity and mortality is added to aggressive management of modifiable risk factors.
> —EXECUTIVE COMMITTEE FOR THE ACAS INVESTIGATORS[1]

Research Question: For patients with asymptomatic carotid stenosis, does carotid endarterectomy (CEA) reduce the 5-year risk of ipsilateral cerebral infarction compared with medical therapy alone?[1]

Funding: National Institute for Neurological Disorders and Stroke. Aspirin was donated by Sterling Health USA.

Year Study Began: 1987

Year Study Published: 1995

Study Location: 39 clinical sites in the United States and Canada.

Who Was Studied: Patients aged 40–79 years with asymptomatic carotid artery stenosis of ≥60% reduction in diameter. The ≥60% stenosis was identified by one of 3 methods: arteriography within the previous 60 days, Doppler ultrasonography, or Doppler ultrasonography plus ocular pneumoplethysmography.

Who Was Excluded: Patients with cerebrovascular events in the distribution of the study carotid artery or in that of the vertebrobasilar arterial system, symptoms referable to the contralateral cerebral hemisphere within the previous 45 days, contraindication to aspirin therapy, a disorder that could seriously complicate surgery, or a condition that could prevent continuing participation or was likely to produce disability or death within 5 years.

How Many Patients: 1,662

Study Overview: See Figure 42.1 for a summary of the study design.

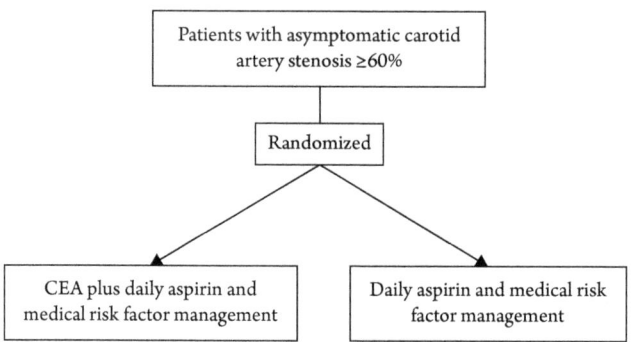

Figure 42.1 Summary of ACAS's Design.

Study Intervention: Patients in both groups received 325 mg daily of regular or enteric-coated aspirin. Stroke risk factors and their modification were reviewed with all patients at the time of randomization and again during subsequent interviews and telephone follow-up. Topics of focus included hypertension, diabetes, lipid management, tobacco cessation, and reducing excessive alcohol consumption. Patients randomized to the surgical arm were scheduled to undergo CEA within 2 weeks of randomization and underwent surgery according to usual protocols.

Follow-Up: Median follow-up was 2.7 years, with 9% of patients completing 5 years of follow-up. The surgeon, the ACAS neurologist, and the ACAS patient coordinator examined each patient 24 hours after CEA. For all patients, follow-up examinations were conducted at 1 month and thereafter every 3 months, alternating between clinic visits and telephone calls. Risk reduction management was reviewed and aspirin adherence was determined by pill count.

Endpoints: Primary outcome: initially, transient ischemic attack (TIA) or cerebral infarction occurring in the distribution of the study artery and any TIA, stroke, or death occurring in the perioperative period. In March 1993, TIA was removed as a primary endpoint, as the ACAS investigators concluded that a recently published trial demonstrated CEA's superiority over medical management in preventing TIA in the setting of asymptomatic carotid stenosis.[2] A TIA was defined as a focal neurological deficit lasting at least 30 seconds and resolving completely within 24 hours. Deficits persisting >24 hours were classified as strokes. Secondary endpoints included any stroke and perioperative death; any stroke and any death; any ipsilateral TIA and stroke; and any perioperative TIA, stroke, or death.

RESULTS

- The estimated 5-year risk of ipsilateral stroke or any perioperative stroke or death was lower in the surgical group vs. the medical therapy group (see Table 42.1).

Table 42.1. SUMMARY OF ACAS'S KEY FINDINGS

Outcome	Estimate of 5-Year Event Risk in Medical Group	Estimate of 5-Year Event Risk in Surgical Group	Reduction Due to Surgery in 5-Year Risk	P Value
Primary outcome: ipsilateral stroke or any perioperative stroke or death	11.0%	5.1%	0.53	0.004
Ipsilateral TIA or stroke or any perioperative TIA or stroke or death	19.2%	8.2%	0.57	<0.001
Any stroke or any perioperative death	17.5%	12.4%	0.29	0.09
Any stroke or death	31.9%	25.6%	0.20	0.08

Criticisms and Limitations: Women and minorities were underrepresented; two-thirds of the patients were men and 95% were white. Women in the study had no significant benefit from surgery. Men benefitted, but mostly those in the 60–69 age range. The perioperative surgical risk was extremely low, <3%. Thus, for these results to be valid, the individual surgeon's operative risk rate must also be <3%. Five of the strokes in the surgical arm were actually caused by preoperative arteriography rather than endarterectomy; these strokes were included in the data and elevated the risk associated with CEA. The overall rates of stroke were very low in general in this trial. The number needed to treat, based on this and other asymptomatic carotid artery surgery trials, is somewhere between 19–50 patients to benefit 1 patient at 5 years. Risk factor modification was not specified, and may not have been aggressive; however, this would hopefully affect both groups similarly. Risk factor modification has evolved greatly since this study was performed, and thus patients treated medically nowadays may have an even more significantly lower risk of stroke or death.

Other Relevant Studies and Information:

- Prior to this study, a Veterans Affairs study[2] demonstrated that CEA significantly reduced the rate of ipsilateral neurological events compared to medical therapy alone in patients with asymptomatic carotid stenosis.
- The Asymptomatic Carotid Surgery Trial (ACST), published in 2004, also demonstrated CEA plus medical management to be superior to medical management alone for 5-year reduction in stroke risk.[3]
- ACST patients were subsequently followed several more years to provide a 10-year estimate of stroke risk following CEA plus medical management versus medical management alone. CEA plus medical management for patients with asymptomatic carotid artery stenosis remained significantly more effective than medical management alone for stroke prevention.[4]
- Guidelines published in 2011 indicate that CEA is reasonable to perform in asymptomatic patients with >70% stenosis of the internal carotid artery if perioperative risk of stroke, myocardial infarction, or death is low.[5]

Summary and Implications: Selected patients with asymptomatic carotid artery stenosis of ≥60% reduction in diameter have a reduced 5-year risk of ipsilateral stroke with CEA plus medical management versus medical management alone. Surgery is associated with perioperative risk, however, and patient preference should be considered when deciding which patients are appropriate candidates for surgery.

CLINICAL CASE: ASYMPTOMATIC CAROTID STENOSIS

Case History:
A 64-year-old man with a history of tobacco abuse and hypertension presented to his primary care doctor's office for a routine evaluation. The exam was noticeable for a bruit over the left carotid artery. The patient denied any recent or remote history of symptoms typically associated with the left carotid artery's distribution, including vision changes or loss, right-sided weakness or sensory changes, or language disturbance. He was subsequently found on duplex ultrasonography to have 80% stenosis of the left proximal internal carotid artery.

Based on the results of this trial, what advice would you give him?

Suggested Answer:
ACAS demonstrated that patients with asymptomatic carotid stenosis >60% reduction in diameter are less likely to have an ipsilateral stroke within 5 years if treated with CEA plus medical management compared to medical management alone. These results were supported in the 5- and 10-year follow-up of patients in the ACST study. Therefore, pursuing CEA is a reasonable choice, if the vascular surgeon's operative morbidity rate is <3%. However, if the patient is anxious about surgical risks, it would also be reasonable for this man to elect for medical therapy.

References

1. Endarterectomy for asymptomatic carotid artery stenosis. Executive Committee for the Asymptomatic Carotid Atherosclerosis Study. *JAMA.* 1995;273(18):1421–1428.
2. Hobson RW, Weiss DG, Fields WS, et al. Efficacy of carotid endarterectomy for asymptomatic carotid stenosis. The Veterans Affairs Cooperative Study Group. *N Engl J Med.* 1993;328(4): 221–227.
3. Halliday A, Mansfield A, Marro J, et al. Prevention of disabling and fatal strokes by successful carotid endarterectomy in patients without recent neurological symptoms: randomised controlled trial. *Lancet.* 2004;363(9420):1491–1502.
4. Halliday A, Harrison M, Hayter E, et al. 10-year stroke prevention after successful carotid endarterectomy for asymptomatic stenosis (ACST-1): a multicentre randomised trial. *Lancet.* 2010;376(9746): 1074–1084.
5. Brott TG, Halperin JL, Abbara S, et al. 2011 ASA/ACCF/AHA/AANN/AANS/ACR/ASNR/CNS/SAIP/SCAI/SIR/SNIS/SVM/SVS guideline on the management of patients with extracranial carotid and vertebral artery disease: a report of the American College of Cardiology Foundation/American Heart Association Task Force on Practice Guidelines, and the American Stroke Association, American

Association of Neuroscience Nurses, American Association of Neurological Surgeons, American College of Radiology, American Society of Neuroradiology, Congress of Neurological Surgeons, Society of Atherosclerosis Imaging and Prevention, Society for Cardiovascular Angiography and Interventions, Society of Interventional Radiology, Society of NeuroInterventional Surgery, Society for Vascular Medicine, and Society for Vascular Surgery. *J Am Coll Cardiol.* 2011;57(8):e16–94.

43

Early Aspirin for Acute Ischemic Stroke
The CAST Trial
MARK LANDRENEAU

... [I]mmediate treatment of acute ischemic stroke with medium dose aspirin produces a modest, but definite net reduction in early death or non-fatal stroke.

—CAST Investigators[1]

Research Question: Is early aspirin use an effective treatment for acute ischemic stroke?[1]

Funding: University of Oxford.

Year Study Began: 1993

Year Study Published: 1997

Study Location: 413 hospitals in China.

Who Was Studied: Patients with suspected ischemic stroke who presented within 48 hours of symptom onset.

Who Was Excluded: Patients with no clear indications for or contraindications to aspirin as determined by the responsible physicians.

How Many Patients: 21,106

Study Overview: See Figure 43.1 for a summary of the study's design.

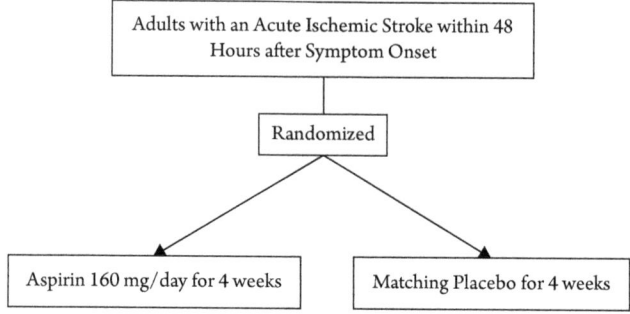

Figure 43.1 Summary of CAST's Design.

Study Intervention: Patients with acute ischemic stroke (symptom onset within 48 hours) were allocated to receive aspirin 160 mg/day for 4 weeks or matching placebo per day for 4 weeks.

Follow-Up: 4 weeks.

Endpoints: Primary outcomes: all-cause mortality during the scheduled treatment period and death or dependent outcome at discharge. Secondary outcomes: fatal or nonfatal recurrent stroke.

RESULTS

- There were 343 (3.3%) in-hospital deaths within 4 weeks among patients allocated aspirin compared with 398 (3.9%) in the placebo group ($P = 0.04$). This correlates to an absolute difference of 5.4 fewer deaths per 1,000 patients.
- There were 335 (3.2%) fatal and nonfatal recurrent strokes among patients allocated aspirin compared to 351 (3.4%) in the placebo group ($P > 0.1$).
- In the aspirin-allocated group, there was an absolute difference of 1.4 more hemorrhagic strokes per 1,000 patients. However, this difference did not reach statistical significance ($P > 0.1$).
- For the combined endpoint of death or nonfatal stroke, there were 545 (5.3%) events in the aspirin group and 614 (5.9%) in the placebo group ($P = 0.03$). This correlates to 6.8 fewer events per 1,000 patients allocated aspirin.

Criticisms and Limitations: Patients were enrolled with *suspected* ischemic stroke, and a CT scan was not required prior to enrollment. A CT scan was only required for comatose patients (87% did receive a scan prior to randomization and nearly all had a CT scan during their hospital stay).

Exclusion criteria were not specified. It was left to the responsible physician to determine if aspirin was safe for each patient, and the responsible physician needed to be uncertain regarding the potential benefit of aspirin. It is unclear how enrolled patients were treated for other comorbidities such as hypertension, diabetes, and smoking, though that may have been mitigated by randomization. The trial also did not include anticoagulation for treatment of patients with atrial fibrillation. Nonetheless, the risk of recurrent stroke for patients with atrial fibrillation in this study was only marginally elevated compared to those who did not have atrial fibrillation.

Other Relevant Studies and Information:

- The International Stroke Trial (IST)[2] was a trial comparable in scope and power (~20,000 patients) that also showed that early aspirin is an effective treatment for acute ischemic stroke in a heterogeneous population.
- A Cochrane Review from 2008[3] supports the use of aspirin for treatment of acute ischemic stroke; over 94% of the data comes from CAST and IST.
- The most recent American Stroke Association guidelines[4] recommend aspirin for the treatment of acute ischemic stroke, though it should not be substituted for other acute interventions such as intravenous recombinant tPA.
- The CHANCE[5] trial has shown that in TIA and minor strokes in a Chinese population, temporary dual antiplatelet therapy with aspirin and clopidogrel may confer greater protection against recurrent ischemic stroke without increasing the risk of hemorrhage.

Summary and Implications: In patients with acute ischemic stroke, a medium dose of aspirin daily is effective at reducing mortality and the risk for recurrent ischemic stroke, though the absolute benefits are modest (6.8 fewer events/ 1,000 patients treated with aspirin).

CLINICAL CASE: ASPIRIN VERSUS PLACEBO FOR ACUTE ISCHEMIC STROKE

Case History:
A 65-year-old woman with hypertension and diabetes presents 12 hours after the acute onset of dysarthria and right-hand weakness. A noncontrast head CT shows a small hypodensity in her left internal capsule without signs of hemorrhage.

Based on the Result of CAST, how should this patient be treated?

Suggested Answer:
CAST showed that medium-dose aspirin (160 mg/day) should be started promptly for patients with acute ischemic stroke and should be continued for at least 4 weeks.

References

1. CAST (Chinese Acute Stroke Trial) Collaborative Group. CAST: randomised placebo controlled trial of early aspirin use in 20 000 patients with acute ischemic stroke. *Lancet.* 1997;349:1641–1649.
2. International Stroke Trial Collaborative Group. The International Stroke Trial (IST): a randomised trial of aspirin, subcutaneous heparin, both, or neither among 19435 patients with acute ischaemic stroke. *Lancet.* 1997;349:1569–1581
3. Sandercock PA, Counsell C, Gubitz GJ, Tseng MC. Antiplatelet therapy for acute ischemic stroke. *Cochrane Database Syst Rev.* 2008;(3):CD000029.
4. Adams HP, del Zoppo G, Alberts MJ, et al. Guidelines for the early management of adults with ischemic stroke. *Stroke.* 2007;38:1655–1711.
5. Wang Y, Wang Y, Zhao X, et al. Clopidogrel with aspirin in acute minor stroke or transient ischemic attack. *N Engl J Med.* 2013;369(1):11–19.

44

Aspirin versus Heparin for Acute Ischemic Stroke

The IST Trial

MARK LANDRENEAU

> Neither heparin regimen offered any clinical advantage at 6 months... For aspirin the IST suggests a small but worthwhile improvement at 6 months.
> —INTERNATIONAL STROKE TRIAL COLLABORATIVE GROUP[1]

Research Question: Is aspirin, heparin, or both an effective therapy in acute ischemic stroke?[1]

Funding: Multiple international organizations. Principally, the International Stroke Trial (IST) was funded by the UK Medical Research Council, UK Stroke Association, and the European BIOMED-1 program.

Year Study Began: 1991

Year Study Published: 1997

Study Location: 467 hospitals in 36 countries.

Who Was Studied: Patients with acute stroke with symptom onset within 48 hours.

Who Was Excluded: Patients with small likelihood of worthwhile benefit (severe preexisting disability or symptoms likely to completely resolve within a few hours); patients with intracranial hemorrhage; patients who had conditions with clear indications or contraindications to aspirin or heparin.

How Many Patients: 19,435

Study Overview: See Figure 44.1 for a summary of the study design.

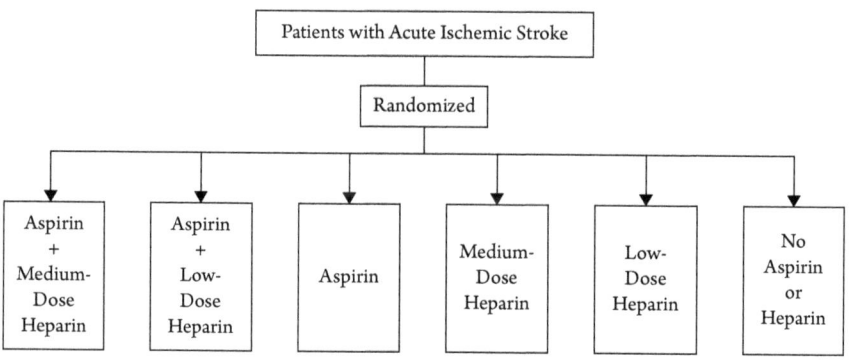

Figure 44.1 Summary of the Trial's Design.

Study Intervention: Patients were randomized to 1 of 6 treatment groups: receiving combination of aspirin 300 mg daily, low-dose heparin (5,000 IU twice daily), medium-dose heparin (12,500 IU twice daily), or nothing. If the patient could not swallow, aspirin was given via nasogastric tube, per rectum, or IV. Patients were treated for 14 days or until discharge. At discharge clinicians were instructed to consider long-term aspirin.

Follow-Up: Follow-up data was collected first at 14 days and again at 6 months.

Endpoints: Primary outcomes: death from any cause within 14 days and death or dependency (defined as needing help from another person with daily activities) at 6 months. Secondary outcomes: symptomatic intracranial hemorrhage within 14 days confirmed by CT, MRI, or autopsy; ischemic stroke within 14 days; major extracranial hemorrhage requiring transfusion or causing death within 14 days; major events within 14 days such as pulmonary embolism; death from any cause at 6 months.

RESULTS

- Patients treated with heparin had fewer recurrent ischemic strokes within 14 days compared to those who "avoided" heparin in the trial, but this benefit was completely offset by an increase in hemorrhagic strokes (see Table 44.1).
- Heparin-treated patients had a significantly high rate of extracranial hemorrhage, corresponding to 9 more hemorrhages per 1,000 patients.
- The negative effect of heparin appeared to be associated with medium-dose heparin, as low-dose heparin was associated with a significant reduction in early death or stroke, corresponding to 12 fewer deaths per 1,000 patients.
- Aspirin-treated patients had a significant reduction in death and stroke, corresponding to 11 fewer events per 1,000 patients, compared to patients who "avoided" aspirin in the trial. At 6 months the aspirin treatment arm had 14 fewer dead or dependent outcomes per 1,000 patients (see Table 44.2).

Table 44.1. SUMMARY OF KEY OUTCOMES AT 14 DAYS

Outcome Events within 14 days	Heparin	No Heparin	Aspirin	No Aspirin
Total deaths	9.0%	9.3%	9.0%	9.4%
Recurrent ischemic stroke	2.9%	3.8%	2.8%	3.9%
Hemorrhagic stroke	1.2%	0.4%	0.9%	0.8%
Extracranial hemorrhage (transfused or fatal)	1.3%	0.4%	1.1%	0.6%

Table 44.2. SUMMARY OF KEY OUTCOMES AT 6 MONTHS

Outcome Events at 6 months	Heparin	No Heparin	Aspirin	No Aspirin
Fully recovered and independent	17.2%	17.0%	17.6%	16.6%
Not recovered but independent	40.4%	41.3%	40.7%	41.0%
Dependent	40.4%	41.3%	40.7%	41.0%
Dead from any cause	22.5%	21.5%	21.5%	22.5%

Criticisms and Limitations: The major criticism of IST is that it was not a placebo-controlled trial. Another study, the Chinese Acute Stroke Trial (CAST) [2] trial, did compare aspirin to a placebo and demonstrated similar rates of risk reduction from aspirin. Furthermore, in IST, in-hospital events were assessed by unblinded clinicians, which could have introduced numerous biases, such as more frequent head CTs for patients on heparin, leading to falsely elevated rates of intracranial hemorrhage simply by more vigilant observation. Only 67% of patients had a CT scan prior to randomization (though an additional 29% had CT scanning shortly after randomization, so, 4% never underwent CT scanning).

Note: a downloadable copy of the full IST dataset is available free of charge for independent analysis.[3]

Other Relevant Studies and Information:

- The CAST trial had similar enrollment numbers as the IST and also showed a significant benefit to the early use of aspirin in the treatment of acute ischemic stroke.
- A Cochrane Review from 2008[4] supports the use of aspirin for acute ischemic stroke, although over 94% of the data come from CAST and IST.
- Another Cochrane Review from 2008[5] based on data of over 16,000 patients combined from multiple trials also supports the use of antiplatelets rather than anticoagulants in the treatment of acute stroke due to the high rates of hemorrhage with unfractionated heparin and low molecular weight heparins. One exception is low-dose heparin combined with aspirin, which may offer a net benefit. Over 80% of that data, however, come from IST.
- The most recent American Stroke Association guidelines[6] recommend antiplatelet therapy—specifically, aspirin for the treatment of acute ischemic stroke, though it should not be substituted for other acute interventions such as intravenous recombinant tPA. Heparin is not recommended as a treatment for acute ischemic stroke.

Summary and Implications: In patients with acute ischemic stroke, aspirin is an effective early treatment to prevent death and disability. Heparin, particularly medium-dose heparin, causes higher rates of hemorrhage that offset any potential benefit. More research is needed to determine whether there may be a role for low-dose heparin, either with or without aspirin, for patients with acute ischemic stroke.

CLINICAL CASE: ASPIRIN VERSUS HEPARIN IN ACUTE ISCHEMIC STROKE

Case History:
A 76-year-old man with a history of hypertension, hyperlipidemia, and coronary artery disease presents 6 hours after the acute onset of confusion and a left visual field cut. He denies any weakness, clumsiness, sensory changes, chest pain, or shortness of breath. On his neurological examination, he is noted to have a left homonymous hemianopsia. His brain MRI demonstrates an area of restricted diffusion in his right occipital lobe without any evidence of hemorrhage.

Based on the results of the IST, should he receive aspirin, heparin, or both for the treatment of his acute stroke?

Suggested Answer:
IST demonstrated that medium-dose heparin was associated with higher rates of intracranial and extracranial hemorrhage that outweigh any potential benefits. This is particularly true for posterior circulation strokes, as they had high rates of hemorrhagic transformation. Daily aspirin was found to be beneficial for acute ischemic stroke, however, and should be instituted immediately. Whether there is a role for low dose heparin, such as is used for venous thromboembolism prophylaxis, requires further study.

References

1. International Stroke Trial Collaborative Group. The International Stroke Trial (IST): a randomised trial of aspirin, subcutaneous heparin, both, or neither among 19435 patients with acute ischaemic stroke. *Lancet*.1997;349:1569–1581.
2. CAST (Chinese Acute Stroke Trial) Collaborative Group. CAST: randomised placebo controlled trial of early aspirin use in 20 000 patients with acute ischemic stroke. *Lancet* 1997;349:1641–1649.
3. Sandercock PAG, Niewada M, Czlonkowska A; The International Stroke Trial database. *Trials*. 2011;12(1):101. http://www.trialsjournal.com/content/12/1/101.
4. Sandercock PA, Counsell C, Gubitz GJ, Tseng MC. Antiplatelet therapy for acute ischemic stroke. *Cochrane Database Syst Rev*. 2008;(3):CD000029.
5. Sandercock PA, Counsell C, Kamal AK. Anticoagulants versus antiplatelet agents for acute ischaemic stroke. *Cochrane Database Syst Rev*. 2008;(4):CD000024.
6. Adams HP, del Zoppo G, Alberts MJ et al. Guidelines for the early management of adults with ischemic stroke. *Stroke*. 2007;38:1655–1711.

45

Dipyridamole and Aspirin for Secondary Stroke Prevention
The ESPS-2 Trial

ROBERT J. CLAYCOMB

> Risk of stroke or death was reduced by 13% with aspirin alone; 15% with dipyridamole alone; and 24% with the combination.
> —Diener et al.[1]

Research Question: The European Stroke Prevention Study (ESPS-1) demonstrated that aspirin 330 mg thrice daily in combination with dipyridamole (a phosphodiesterase inhibitor) 75 mg thrice daily significantly reduced the incidence of stroke in those patients with a previous transient ischemic attack (TIA) or a previous stroke.[2] However, the higher doses of aspirin may have increased risk of bleeding.[3] This study asked: how do placebo, low-dose aspirin alone, dipyridamole alone, and the combination of aspirin and dipyridamole compare with regard to secondary stroke prevention and bleeding risk?[1]

Funding: Supported by a grant from Boehringer Ingelheim.

Year Study Began: 1989

Year Study Published: 1995

Study Location: 59 sites within 13 European countries.

Who Was Studied: Patients who were aged ≥18 years and had either a TIA or confirmed ischemic stroke within the previous 3 months were included in the study.

Who Was Excluded: Patients were excluded if they had any of the following: (1) peptic ulcer disease; (2) previous gastrointestinal bleeding; (3) hypersensitivity to aspirin or dipyridamole; (4) bleeding disorder; (5) any condition requiring continued use of aspirin or anticoagulants; or (6) any life-threatening condition.

How Many Patients: 6,602

Study Overview: See Figure 45.1 for a summary of the study design.

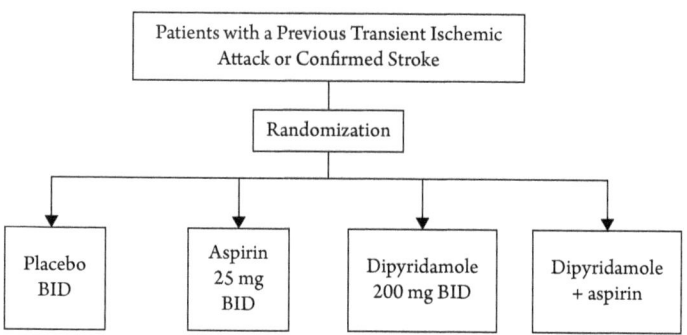

Figure 45.1 Summary of ESPS-2's Design.

Study Intervention: Patients were randomized to receive either: (1) placebo twice daily; (2) aspirin 25 mg twice daily; (3) modified-release dipyridamole 200 mg twice daily; or (4) aspirin 25 mg and extended-release dipyridamole 200 mg twice daily.

Follow-Up: 2 years. One follow-up visit conducted at 1 month, and then follow-up visits every 3 months until trial completion.

Endpoints: Primary endpoints were the incidence of stroke and/or death. Secondary endpoints were TIA, myocardial infarction, other ischemic events, and other vascular events.

RESULTS

- "Stroke risk was significantly reduced by 18.1% (p = 0.013) with aspirin alone, by 16.3% (p = 0.039) with dipyridamole alone, and by 37.0% (p < 0.0010 with combination therapy, when compared to placebo)" (see Table 45.1).[1]
- None of the treatments reduced the risk of death relative to placebo.
- There was a statistically significant decrease in other vascular events (pulmonary embolism, deep venous thrombosis, peripheral artery obstruction, and retinal artery occlusion) associated with antiplatelet treatments.
- Rates of bleeding were nearly 2 times greater in patients receiving aspirin-containing therapies relative to placebo; however, there was no increase in bleeding rates with dipyridamole alone.
- Nearly 4 times as many patients who were receiving dipyridamole-containing treatments (265, 4.0%) self-discontinued their medications due to headache versus those receiving therapies without dipyridamole (70, 1.1%).

Table 45.1. SUMMARY OF ESPS-2'S KEY FINDINGS[a]

Outcome after 24 months	Placebo	Aspirin Alone	Dipyridamole Alone	Dipyridamole and Aspirin
Stroke	15.8%	12.9%	13.2%	9.9%
Stroke or Death	22.9%	20.0%	19.4%	17.3%

[a] Values are percentages of patients with the indication outcome for each of the treatments.

Criticisms and Limitations:

- There was no strategy in place to deal with patients who developed headache.[4]
- This study used an unusual aspirin dosing schedule; the more standard aspirin dose of aspirin is 81 mg daily. However, this dose was employed because the investigators wanted a low dose of aspirin given the results of previous trials[5,6] and 81 mg aspirin was not available in Europe.[4] Also, pharmacological data indicated that the best ratio between dipyridamole and aspirin was 8:1.[4] Therefore if a higher dose of aspirin was used, a higher dose of dipyridamole would need to be used, which would have increased the risk of side effects such as headache.[4]

- The formulation of dipyridamole was different from the immediate-release form studied in ESPS-1[2], which required being taken at least thrice daily, impacting compliance. The extended-release formulation used in ESPS-2 is administered twice daily, aiding in patient compliance, and achieving more consistent serum levels.
- At the time the study was published, some reviewers thought the inclusion of a placebo arm was unethical and refused publication, despite the study's approval from 59 different institutional review boards.[7] However, at the time of the study there were no single placebo-controlled trials that demonstrated superiority for aspirin after stroke prevention as the primary endpoint.[4] Also, it was only after the results of the ESPS2 study that aspirin was approved for secondary stroke prevention.
- ESPS2 was one of the first trials with monitoring that was able to expose 1 center that falsified data.[4] The results from that center were excluded from the analysis, and thus did not affect the results.

Other Relevant Studies and Information:

- The academically driven ESPRIT study also compared the efficacy of aspirin and dipyridamole and demonstrated that the combination of the 2 medications was associated with a decreased relative risk of stroke over 3.5 years (13% and 16% for aspirin and aspirin + dipyridamole, respectively).[8]
- The PRoFESS study compared the efficacy of the aspirin-dipyridamole combination with clopidogrel for secondary stroke prevention and found no difference between the two antiplatelet agents.[9] This study, in combination with a specific subgroup analysis of the CAPRIE study[10] that did not find a significant difference between aspirin alone and clopidogrel alone for secondary stroke prevention, has led to relative equipoise with regards to antiplatelet therapy selection for patients after stroke. However, it should be noted that the PRoFESS trial included a disproportionate number of strokes secondary to small vessel disease, leading to slower than expected event rates and may have impacted the results.
- Of note, both aspirin-dipyridamole and clopidogrel are more expensive options compared with aspirin.
- The 2014 guidelines from the American Heart Association and the American Stroke Association state that "aspirin (50–325 mg/d) monotherapy or the combination of aspirin 25 mg and extended-release dipyridamole 200 mg twice daily is indicated as initial therapy after TIA or ischemic stroke for prevention of future stroke."[11] Also, "clopidogrel

(75 mg) monotherapy is a reasonable option for secondary prevention of stroke in place of aspirin or combination aspirin/dipyridamole."[11]

Summary and Implications: The ESPS-2 study demonstrated that for secondary stroke prevention, the combination of low-dose aspirin (25 mg twice a day) and extended-release dipyridamole (200 mg twice a day) is associated with a decreased risk of stroke, and that this reduction is greater than for either drug alone. Combination therapy with aspirin and extended-release dipyridamole is now recommended as a first-line antiplatelet agent regimen for secondary stroke prevention (clopidogrel is also considered to be a first-line agent for secondary stroke prevention [especially in patients with an aspirin allergy], and aspirin monotherapy is also appropriate if there are financial barriers to the other therapies).

CLINICAL CASE: ASPIRIN AND DIPYRIDAMOLE FOR SECONDARY STROKE PREVENTION

Case History:
A 63-year-old woman with a history of a previous left subcortical lacunar infarct, hypertension, hyperlipidemia, diabetes mellitus, and chronic daily headaches presents for routine posthospitalization follow-up after her stroke. During her hospitalization she was started on aspirin 81 mg daily. Her extended cardiac monitoring revealed no evidence of paroxysmal atrial fibrillation. She has no clinical history of heart failure and no history of hemorrhage or bleeding diathesis. She takes an angiotensin-converting enzyme inhibitor, a statin, thrice daily insulin, and topiramate for her headaches.

Her exam is notable for mild hemiparesis of her right leg and she walks with a cane. Routine lab work was completely unremarkable. An MRI of her brain reveals chronic microvascular disease and confirms her prior stroke.

Should this patient be treated with aspirin and extended-release dipyridamole?

Suggested Answer:
Likely not. This patient has a clear indication for an antiplatelet agent such as aspirin or dipyridamole and no compelling indication for anticoagulation. Given her history of chronic daily headaches that require topiramate, it is likely that she would not be able to tolerate dipyridamole. Moreover, if the dipyridamole were combined with aspirin in a single capsule (as is commonly done) and she stopped taking the combination medication due to her headaches, she would risk being completely without antiplatelet therapy. Continuing aspirin 81 mg daily is a reasonable option for her.

References

1. Diener HC, Cunha L, Forbes C, Sivenius J, Smets P, Lowenthal A. European Stroke Prevention Study. 2. Dipyridamole and acetylsalicylic acid in the secondary prevention of stroke. *J Neurol Sci.* 1996;143(1-2):1–13.
2. The European Stroke Prevention Study (ESPS). Principal end-points. The ESPS Group. *Lancet.* 1987;2(8572):1351–1354.
3. Collaborative overview of randomised trials of antiplatelet therapy—III: Reduction in venous thrombosis and pulmonary embolism by antiplatelet prophylaxis among surgical and medical patients. Antiplatelet Trialists' Collaboration. *BMJ.* 1994;308(6923):235–246.
4. Personal communication from Dr. Diener.
5. A comparison of two doses of aspirin (30 mg vs. 283 mg a day) in patients after a transient ischemic attack or minor ischemic stroke. The Dutch TIA Trial Study Group. *N Engl J Med.* 1991;325(18):1261–1266.
6. Swedish Aspirin Low-Dose Trial (SALT) of 75 mg aspirin as secondary prophylaxis after cerebrovascular ischaemic events. The SALT Collaborative Group. *Lancet.* 1991;338(8779):1345–1349.
7. Diener HC. How much esprit is in ESPRIT? *Stroke.* 2006;37(11): 2856–2857.
8. Halkes et al., Aspirin plus dipyridamole versus aspirin alone after cerebral ischaemia of arterial origin (ESPRIT): randomised controlled trial. *Lancet.* 2006;367(9523):1665–1673.
9. Sacco RL, Diener HC, Yusuf S, et al. Aspirin and extended-release dipyridamole versus clopidogrel for recurrent stroke. *N Engl J Med.* 2008;359(12):1238–1251.
10. A randomised, blinded, trial of clopidogrel versus aspirin in patients at risk of ischaemic events (CAPRIE). CAPRIE Steering Committee. *Lancet.* 1996;348(9038);1329–1339.
11. Kernan WN, Ovbiagele B, Black HR, et al. Guidelines for the prevention of stroke in patients with stroke and transient ischemic attack: a guideline for healthcare professionals from the American Heart Association/American Stroke Association. *Stroke.* 2014;45:2160–2236.

46

High-Dose Atorvastatin after Stroke or Transient Ischemic Attack

The SPARCL Trial

BRIAN MAC GRORY

> ... in patients with a recent stroke or TIA, treatment with 80 mg of atorvastatin per day decreased the risk of stroke, major coronary events, and revascularization procedures.
>
> —The SPARCL Investigators[1]

Research Question: Is there evidence that a daily dose of 80 mg atorvastatin reduces the risk of stroke in patients with no known coronary heart disease who have had a stroke or transient ischemic attack (TIA) within the previous 6 months?[1]

Funding: Pfizer.

Year Study Began: 1998

Year Study Published: 2006

Study Location: 205 medical centers predominantly in the United States, Europe, and Australia.

Who Was Studied: Patients aged >18 with a history of (1) ischemic stroke, (2) hemorrhagic stroke, or (3) TIA between 1–6 months prior to randomization.

Who Was Excluded: Patients with atrial fibrillation, cardioembolic stroke, or subarachnoid hemorrhage. Also excluded were patients who were not ambulatory, had a modified Rankin Score >3 or LDL <100mg/dL.

How Many Patients: 4,731

Study Overview: See Figure 46.1 for a summary of the study design.

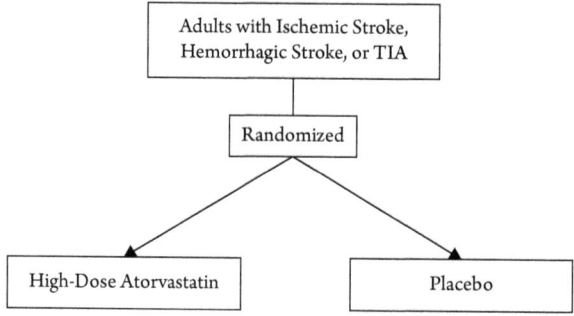

Figure 46.1 Summary of SPARCL's Design.

Study Intervention: Eligible patients were randomly assigned to receive 80 mg atorvastatin per day or placebo.

Follow-Up: Median of 4.9 years. Follow-up visits were scheduled 1, 3, and 6 months after enrollment and every 6 months thereafter.

Endpoints: Primary outcome was time from randomization to first stroke. Secondary outcomes were stroke/TIA, major coronary events, major cardiovascular event (defined as stroke as well as a major coronary event, any coronary events, revascularization procedure, and any cardiovascular event—i.e., any of the previous 6 criteria in the context of symptomatic peripheral vascular disease).

RESULTS

- A total of 6,670 patients were selected for screening, of whom 4,731 ultimately underwent randomization: 2,365 were then assigned to receive 80 mg atorvastatin per day and 2,366 to receive a placebo. Of these, 2,272 patients in the intervention group were followed until the end of the study, and 2,253 patients from the placebo group were followed until the end of the study. All randomized patients were included in the final analysis, however.
- Mean LDL levels were similar in the 2 groups at baseline. By 1 month into the trial, LDL in the atorvastatin group had fallen by 53% compared with no change in the placebo group ($P < 0.001$).
- Mean LDL levels in the treatment group were 72.9 mg/dL versus 128.5 mg/dL in the placebo group ($P < 0.001$). Total cholesterol levels in the treatment group were 147.2 mg/dL versus 208.4 mg/dL in the control group.
- The primary endpoint was observed in 265 patients in the treatment group versus 311 in the placebo group.
- Absolute difference in mortality from stroke between the 2 groups was 2.2% (with a 95% confidence interval of 0.2%–4.2%).
- Atorvastatin was associated with a 16% relative reduction in the risk of stroke ($P = 0.03$).
- There were reductions in the combined risk of stroke/TIA and the risk of major coronary events in the treatment arm of the study.
- There was no difference in overall mortality between the 2 groups.
- There was an increase in the risk of hemorrhagic stroke in the atorvastatin group (with a cause-specific adjusted hazard ratio of 1.66).

Criticisms and Limitations:

- The investigators did not gather data on the level of disability arising from strokes in the respective groups. This information is important as the most important effect of stroke on a population is the increased burden of disability as opposed to mortality.
- Although mortality from cerebrovascular and cardiovascular disease was reduced in the treatment group, overall mortality between the 2 groups did not differ which might suggest that the study was

underpowered. This trial specifically dealt with patients without atrial fibrillation and without a history of coronary artery disease. This makes its results difficult to generalize to the population at large.
- The authors did not report on the incidence of myalgias, which are known to occur commonly in patients on statins, often leading to their discontinuation.
- There was no breakdown by stroke subtype; it is unclear whether patients without atherosclerotic disease (e.g., dissection or small vessel disease) have the same benefit from statins.
- The absolute risk reduction was 2.2% over 5 years, or less than 0.5% per year on average. Furthermore, the benefit from being on a statin only appeared after prolonged use.
- All of the authors had financial conflicts of interest in the form of a relationship with the sponsoring pharmaceutical company, Pfizer.

Other Relevant Studies and Information:

- A secondary analysis of the data from the SPARCL trial that specifically concerned those patients enrolled who had type 2 diabetes mellitus found that statins had no benefit in this population.[2]
- A multicenter study, the Thrombolysis and Statins (THRaST) trial, of the use of statins used in the acute phase of stroke (immediately post-thrombolysis) found a beneficial effect in terms of improved functional outcome and reduced risk of mortality.[3]
- Elkind et al.[4] reported an observational study on the effects of being on a statin prior to having an acute ischemic stroke. They found that patients already taking a statin who have an acute ischemic stroke have a lower poststroke mortality (at 90 days) and a reduced risk of deterioration during their hospitalization.

Summary and Implications: In patients with a history of stroke or TIA within the past 6 months, 80 mg of atorvastatin per day reduced the risk of subsequent stroke in patients without known coronary artery disease. There was an associated reduction in the LDL and total cholesterol levels in the treatment group versus the placebo group. The number needed to treat for five years was 46 to eliminate 1 stroke.

CLINICAL CASE: THE USE OF LIPID-LOWERING THERAPY AFTER ACUTE ISCHEMIC STROKE

Case History:
A 73-year-old gentleman with a background of hypertension and hyperlipidemia is being seen in follow-up with his primary care physician after being hospitalized for an acute ischemic stroke felt to be due to small vessel disease in the context of poorly managed vascular risk factors. He has no residual deficits from his stroke and is independent in all his basic and instrumental activities of daily living. He has no known history of coronary artery disease. His LDL cholesterol is measured at 155 mg/dL.

What are the beneficial effects for this man of using statin therapy as a lipid-lowering agent?

Suggested Answer:
The SPARCL trial suggested that there was a reduction in overall mortality from stroke in patients treated with 80 mg of atorvastatin per day (in a population without known coronary artery disease or atrial fibrillation). Atorvastatin was also associated with a 16% reduced risk of further ischemic stroke at the cost of a slightly elevated risk of hemorrhagic stroke. It would therefore be reasonable to recommend it to this gentleman as part of ongoing secondary prevention of further cerebrovascular events.

References

1. Amarenco P, Bogousslavsky J, Callahan A, et al. High-dose atorvastatin after stroke or transient ischemic attack. *N Engl J Med*. 2006;355(6):549–559.
2. Callahan A, Amarenco P, Goldstein LB, et al. Risk of stroke and cardiovascular events after ischemic stroke or transient ischemic attack in patients with type 2 diabetes or metabolic syndrome: secondary analysis of the Stroke Prevention by Aggressive Reduction in Cholesterol Levels (SPARCL) trial. *Arch Neurol*. 2011;68(10):1245–1251.
3. Cappellari M, Bovi P, Moretto G, et al. The THRombolysis and STatins (THRaST) study. *Neurology*. 2013;80(7):655–661.
4. Elkind MS, Flint AC, Sciacca RR, Sacco RL. Lipid-lowering agent use at ischemic stroke onset is associated with decreased mortality. *Neurology*. 2005;65(2):253–258.

47

Adjusted-Dose Warfarin for Stroke Prevention in High-Risk Atrial Fibrillation Patients
The SPAF III Trial

DANIEL C. BROOKS

> Low-intensity, fixed-dose warfarin plus aspirin . . . is insufficient for stroke prevention in patients with non-valvular [atrial fibrillation] at high-risk for thromboembolism; adjusted-dose warfarin . . . reduces stroke for high-risk patients.
> —The SPAF III Investigators[1]

Research Question: Is the combination of aspirin and low-intensity, fixed-dose warfarin (a) as efficacious and (b) safer than adjusted-dose warfarin in the prevention of stroke in patients with atrial fibrillation?[1]

Funding: The trial was supported by a grant from the Division of Stroke and Trauma, National Institute for Neurological Disorders and Stroke. Warfarin was donated by DuPont-Merck Pharma. Aspirin was donated by SmithKline Beecham Consumer Brands.

Year Study Began: 1993

Year Study Published: 1996

Study Location: 20 clinical sites in the United States and Canada

Who Was Studied: Adults with atrial fibrillation documented in the 6 months preceding the study plus one or more of the following characteristics: impaired left ventricular function (congestive heart failure within the previous 100 days or fractional shortening <25%); systolic blood pressure >160 at study entry; prior ischemic stroke, transient ischemic attack (TIA), or systemic embolism; or female aged >75 years. Patients who had had a nondisabling stroke or TIA were eligible 30 days poststroke/TIA.

Who Was Excluded: Patients with prosthetic heart valves, mitral stenosis, or other conditions such as recent pulmonary embolism that required anticoagulation, or contraindications to aspirin or warfarin.

How Many Patients: 1,044

Study Overview: See Figure 47.1 for a summary of the study design.

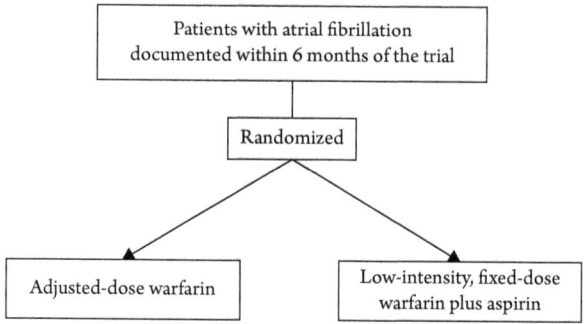

Figure 47.1 Summary of SPAF III's Design.

Study Intervention: Patients in the adjusted-dose warfarin group received an initial dose based on age, followed by weekly international normalized ratio (INR) measurements with dose adjustments until stabilized within the INR range of 2.0–3.0. These patients were monitored at least monthly after this. Patients in the low-intensity, fixed-dose warfarin plus aspirin group received warfarin to raise the INR between 1.2–1.5 on 2 successive measurements 1 week apart; then their INRs were monitored after 1 month, after 3 months, and then every 3 months. If the INR exceeded 3.0 or if bleeding occurred, the fixed dose was reduced. These patients also received aspirin 325 mg daily.

Follow-Up: Mean of 1.1 years

Endpoints: Primary outcome: the rate of ischemic stroke and systemic embolism. Secondary outcomes: TIA, disabling or fatal stroke, major hemorrhage, and a composite of primary events or vascular death.

RESULTS

- The trial was stopped early after a mean follow-up of 1.1 years.
- The rate of primary events (ischemic stroke or systemic embolism) in patients receiving combination therapy was significantly greater than in those receiving adjusted-dose warfarin (see Table 47.1).
- Adjusted-dose warfarin was associated with significantly fewer disabling strokes compared to combination therapy (see Table 47.1).
- Rates of major hemorrhage did not differ significantly between the groups (see Table 47.1).

Table 47.1. SUMMARY OF SPAF III's KEY FINDINGS

Outcome	Adjusted-dose Warfarin (n = 523)	Fixed-dose Warfarin plus Aspirin (n = 521)	Absolute Rate Difference	P Value
Total primary events (ischemic stroke or systemic embolism)	1.9%	7.9%	6.0%	<0.0001
Transient ischemic attack	2.7%	4.5%		NS
All disabling/fatal strokes	1.7%	5.6%	3.9%	0.0007
Major hemorrhage (includes intracranial hemorrhage)	2.1%	2.4%		NS
Primary event or vascular death	6.4%	11.8%	5.4%	0.002

Criticisms and Limitations: The medications were given open label, although assessment of endpoints was done in a blinded fashion. Early termination of the trial may have exaggerated differences between the groups. A 1-year follow up period may not have been sufficient, and long-term safety could not be assessed. The comparison of adjusted-dose warfarin was to a combination of medications uncommonly used (low-intensity warfarin therapy in addition to aspirin).

Other Relevant Studies and Information:

- The ACTIVE W trial in 2006[2] demonstrated the superiority of warfarin versus aspirin plus clopidogrel for the reduction of stroke risk in patients with atrial fibrillation.
- More than a decade after this study was published, three newer oral anticoagulants (dabigatran, rivaroxaban, and apixaban) have been compared to adjusted-dose warfarin for the prevention of stroke in atrial fibrillation. All three studies indicate that adjusted-dose warfarin remains highly efficacious.[3-5]
- Warfarin remains first-line therapy for the prevention of stroke in atrial fibrillation in guidelines published by the American Academy of Neurology[6] and the American College of Cardiology/American Heart Association.[7]

Summary and Implications: Adjusted-dose warfarin with a target INR of 2.0–3.0 is more efficacious than low-intensity, fixed-dose warfarin plus aspirin in preventing stroke in patients with atrial fibrillation. Major bleeding rates were similar between groups.

CLINICAL CASE: STROKE PREVENTION IN ATRIAL FIBRILLATION

A 77-year-old woman with atrial fibrillation and a history of nondisabling stroke, with no vascular events in over 2 years since starting warfarin, presented to her primary care doctor's office to inquire about discontinuing warfarin, or at least decreasing the dose, so that she would not need to have her INR checked very often. She offered to take aspirin instead.

Based on the results of this trial, what advice would you give her?

Suggested Answer:
SPAF III demonstrated the superiority of warfarin versus aspirin plus low-intensity, fixed-dose warfarin for stroke prevention in atrial fibrillation. A subsequent study, ACTIVE W, revealed warfarin to also be superior to dual antiplatelet therapy with aspirin plus clopidogrel. Her $CHADS_2$ score is 3, which is similar to the patient profile in the ROCKET AF trial. Since she has done well so far on warfarin, it might be advisable to continue with the current regimen; however, if she feels strongly that she does not want to continue the frequent monitoring, it would also be reasonable to discuss with her the risks and benefits of the newer anticoagulants that do not require regular anticoagulation testing.

References

1. Adjusted-dose warfarin versus low-intensity, fixed-dose warfarin plus aspirin for high-risk patients with atrial fibrillation: Stroke Prevention in Atrial Fibrillation III randomised clinical trial. *Lancet*. 1996;348(9028):633–638.
2. Connolly S, Pogue J, Hart R, et al., Clopidogrel plus aspirin versus oral anticoagulation for atrial fibrillation in the Atrial fibrillation Clopidogrel Trial with Irbesartan for prevention of Vascular Events (ACTIVE W): a randomised controlled trial. *Lancet*. 2006;367(9526):1903–1912.
3. Connolly SJ, Ezekowitz MD, Yusuf S, et al. Dabigatran versus warfarin in patients with atrial fibrillation. *N Engl J Med*. 2009;361(12):1139–1151.
4. Patel MR, Mahaffey KW, Garg J, et al. Rivaroxaban versus warfarin in nonvalvular atrial fibrillation. *N Engl J Med*. 2011;365(10):883–891.
5. Granger, CB, Alexander JH, McMurray JJV et al. Apixaban versus warfarin in patients with atrial fibrillation. *N Engl J Med*. 2011;365(11):981–992.
6. Culebras A, Messé SR, Chaturvedi S, Kase CS, Gronseth G. Summary of evidence-based guideline update: prevention of stroke in nonvalvular atrial fibrillation: report of the Guideline Development Subcommittee of the American Academy of Neurology. *Neurology*. 2014;82(8):716–724.
7. January CT, Wann S, Alpert JS, et al. 2014 AHA/ACC/HRS guideline for the management of patients with atrial fibrillation: a report of the American College of Cardiology/American Heart Association Task Force on practice guidelines and the Heart Rhythm Society. *Circulation*. 2014;130(23):e199–267.

Dabigatran for Stroke Prevention in Atrial Fibrillation Patients

The RE-LY Trial

ROBERT J. CLAYCOMB

> ... dabigatran given at a dose of 110 mg was associated with rates of stroke and systemic embolism that were similar to those associated with warfarin...
>
> —CONNOLLY ET AL.[1]

Research Question: How does dabigatran, a direct thrombin inhibitor, compare to adjusted-dose warfarin for risk reduction of stroke in patients with atrial fibrillation?[1]

Funding: Supported by a grant from Boehringer Ingelheim Pharmaceuticals.

Year Study Began: 2005

Year Study Published: 2009

Study Location: 951 clinical centers in 44 countries in Asia, Europe, North America, and South America.

Who Was Studied: Patients who had documented atrial fibrillation and at least one of the following: (1) "a previous stroke or transient ischemic attack"; (2) "a left ventricular ejection fraction of less than 40%"; (3) "New York Heart Association class II or higher heart-failure symptoms within 6 month of study inclusion"; (4) "age greater than 75"; or (5) age between 65–74 with hypertension, diabetes mellitus, or coronary artery disease.[1]

Who Was Excluded: Patients were excluded if they had any of the following: (1) "severe heart valve disorder," (2) "stroke within 14 days of inclusion," (3) "severe stroke within 6 months of inclusion," (4) "a condition that increased the risk of hemorrhage," (5) "a creatinine clearance of less than 30mL per minute," (6) "active liver disease," or (7) "pregnancy."[1]

How Many Patients: 18,133

Study Overview: See Figure 48.1 for a summary of the study design.

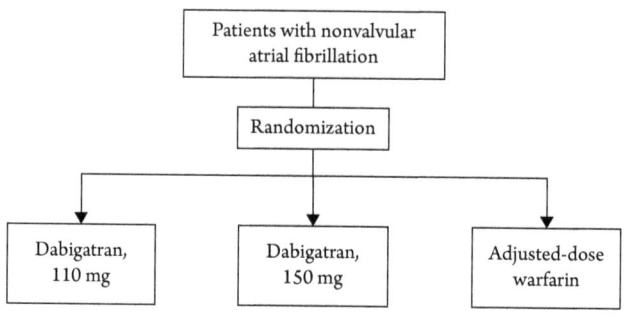

Figure 48.1 Summary of Study Design.

Study Intervention: Patients were randomized to receive either dabigatran 110 mg twice a day, 150 mg twice a day, or adjusted-dose warfarin daily. Patients receiving warfarin had their doses adjusted to achieve an international normalized ratio (INR) of 2.0–3.0, and this was assessed at least monthly. The patients receiving dabigatran did not have any routine monitoring of their INR or coagulation status. Regardless of treatment, all patients had routine monitoring of liver function tests and routine follow-up visits at "14 days after randomization, at 1 and 3 months, every 3 months thereafter in the first year, and then every 4 months until the study ended."[1]

Follow-Up: 2 years.

Endpoints: Primary outcomes: stroke or systemic embolism. The primary safety outcome was major bleeding as defined as "a reduction of the hemoglobin by at least 20 g per liter, transfusion of at least 2 units of blood, or symptomatic bleeding in a critical area or organ."[1] Other outcomes: (1) life-threatening bleeding (a subcategory of major bleeding) defined by either "fatal bleeding, symptomatic intracranial bleeding, bleeding with a decrease in the hemoglobin concentration of at least 50 g per liter, bleeding requiring a transfusion of 4 or more units of blood, use of inotropic agents due to bleeding or bleeding requiring surgery"[1]; (2) incidence of myocardial infarction; (3) pulmonary embolism; (4) transient ischemic attack; or (5) hospitalization.

RESULTS

- "Both dabigatran doses were non-inferior to warfarin"[1] (Table 48.1). "The 150 mg dose of dabigatran was superior to warfarin with respect to stroke or systemic embolism" [1] (Table 48.1). "The 110 mg dose [of dabigatran] was superior to warfarin with respect to major bleeding"[1] (Table 48.2). There was no statistically significant difference with respect to major bleeding between dabigatran 150 mg and warfarin. (Table 48.2).
- Although there was no statistically significant difference in the incidence of pulmonary embolism within the three groups, patients receiving dabigatran 150 mg twice a day had a statistically significant greater increase of myocardial infarction (0.74% vs. 0.53%) as compared to those on warfarin therapy.
- The net clinical benefit outcome was calculated which compared the composite of stroke, systemic embolism, pulmonary embolism, myocardial infarction, death, and major bleeding between the three groups. It was determined that dabigatran 150 mg had a statistically significant decrease in the composite of the aforementioned events as compared to warfarin (6.91% vs. 7.64%, $P = 0.04$, for dabigatran 150 mg and warfarin, respectively).
- The rates of patient-initiated discontinuation of therapy were similar between patients taking dabigatran 100 mg (7.3%), 150 mg (7.8%), and adjusted-dose warfarin (6.2%), despite the fact warfarin users needed frequent coagulation testing.
- The incidence of dyspepsia was statistically increased in both dabigatran groups as compared to warfarin-treated patients (11.8%, 11.3%, and 5.8% for dabigatran 110 mg and 150 mg and warfarin, respectively).

Table 48.1. SUMMARY OF KEY FINDINGS

Event	Dabigatran Dosage[a]		Adjusted-Dose Warfarin[a]	P VALUES FOR DABIGATRAN COMPARISON		
	110 mg	150 mg		110 mg vs. Warfarin	150 mg vs. Warfarin	150 mg vs. 110 mg
Stroke or systemic embolism	1.53%	1.11%	1.69%	<0.001[b]	<0.001[b]	0.005
Hemorrhagic stroke	0.12%	0.10%	0.38%	<0.001	<0.001	0.67
Ischemic or unspecified stroke	1.34%	0.92%	1.20%	0.35	0.03	0.002
Disabling or fatal stroke	0.94%	0.66%	1.00%	0.65	0.005	0.02
Death from vascular causes	2.43%	2.28%	2.69%	0.21	0.04	0.44

[a] Values are number of patients, percent per patient year.
[b] P value for noninferiority, all others P values calculated for superiority.

Table 48.2. HEMORRHAGIC EVENTS

Type of Hemorrhage	Dabigatran Dosage[a]		Adjusted-Dose Warfarin[a]	P VALUES FOR DABIGATRAN COMPARISON		
	110 mg	150 mg		110 mg vs. Warfarin	150 mg vs. Warfarin	150 mg vs. 110 mg
Major bleeding	2.71%	3.11%	3.36	0.003	0.31	0.052
Major or minor bleeding	14.62%	16.42%	18.15%	<0.001	0.002	<0.001
Life-threatening bleeding	1.22%	1.45%	1.80%	<0.001	0.04	0.11
Intracranial bleeding	0.23%	0.30%	0.74%	<0.001	<0.001	0.28
Gastrointestinal bleeding	1.12%	1.51%	1.02%	0.43	<0.001	0.007

[a] Values are number of patients, percent per patient year.

Criticisms and Limitations: The use of aspirin was allowed in approximately 40% of all groups. Concurrent use of aspirin and oral anticoagulants has been shown to increase bleeding risk and likely increased the incidence of major bleeding in all groups.[1]

At the time of the study, there was no well-established antidote or reversal agent for dabigatran in the setting of life-threatening hemorrhage, while warfarin-reversal is commonplace.

The safety of direct thrombin inhibitors in the setting of renal insufficiency, including the elderly, is not well established.

Other Relevant Studies and Information:

- Longer-term follow up of the RE-LY study (RELY-ABLE) confirmed both the safety and efficacy of dabigatran and indicated that the higher dose of dabigatran (150 mg) was associated with a higher rate of bleeding versus the lower dose (110 mg).[3]
- The American Academy of Neurology recognized dabigatran as a viable alternative to warfarin therapy in patients with nonvalvular atrial fibrillation in their latest practice guidelines.[4]

Summary and Implications: This study demonstrated that dabigatran 110 mg and 150 mg are not inferior to adjusted-dose warfarin for the prevention of stroke and systemic embolism in patients with nonvalvular atrial fibrillation. Dabigatran may be a viable alternative to adjusted-dose warfarin, which does not require anticoagulation monitoring.

CLINICAL CASE: DABIGATRAN FROM STROKE PREVENTION IN NONVALVULAR ATRIAL FIBRILLATION

Case History:

A 77-year-old man with a history of a previous right middle cerebral artery stroke and hypertension presents for follow-up after extended cardiac monitoring (performed to determine the etiology of his stroke) revealed paroxysmal atrial fibrillation. He has no clinical history of heart failure and no history of hemorrhage or bleeding diathesis.

His exam is notable for mild paresis of his left arm, but is otherwise unremarkable, including no gait disturbance. Routine lab work revealed a normal creatinine clearance and no evidence of coagulopathy. A recent routine stress test revealed no evidence of coronary artery disease. His cardiac echocardiogram demonstrated no evidence of valvular abnormalities and a normal left systolic ejection fraction. An MRI of his brain reveals several T2-hyperintense lesions consistent with multiple previous cardioembolic strokes but no new strokes and no evidence of previous hemorrhage.

Should this patient be treated with dabigatran for secondary stroke prevention?

Suggested Answer:

Yes. Dabigatran is a viable alternative to warfarin therapy in this patient who would benefit from anticoagulation. There are no contraindications to dabigatran in this patient, and he would not require any anticoagulation monitoring.

References

1. Connolly JS, Ezekowitz MD, Yusuf S, et al. Dabigatran versus warfarin in patients with atrial fibrillation. *N Engl J Med.* 2009;361(12):1139–1151.
2. Lechat P, Lardoux H, Mallet A, et al. Anticoagulant (fluindione)-aspirin combination in patients with high-risk atrial fibrillation. A randomized trial (Fluindione, Fibrillation Auriculaire, Aspirin et Contraste Spontané; FFAACS). *Cerebrovasc Dis.* 2001;12:245–252.
3. Connolly SJ, Wallentin L, Ezekowitz MD, et al. The long-term multicenter observational study of dabigatran treatment in patients with atrial fibrillation (RELY-ABLE) study. *Circulation.* 2013;128:237–243.
4. Culebras A, Messé SR, Chaturvedi S, Kase CS, Gronseth G. Summary of evidence-based guideline update: prevention of stroke in nonvalvular atrial fibrillation: report of the Guideline Development Subcommittee of the American Academy of Neurology. *Neurology.* 2014;82:716–724.

Apixaban for Stroke Prevention in Atrial Fibrillation Patients

The ARISTOTLE Trial

DANIEL C. BROOKS

In patients with atrial fibrillation, apixaban was superior to warfarin in preventing stroke or systemic embolism, caused less bleeding, and resulted in lower mortality.
—GRANGER ET AL.[1]

Research Question: How does the oral factor Xa inhibitor apixaban compare to warfarin in patients with atrial fibrillation in (a) preventing ischemic or hemorrhagic stroke or systemic embolism and (b) its association with major bleeding and death from any cause?[1]

Funding: Bristol-Myers Squibb and Pfizer.

Year Study Began: 2006

Year Study Published: 2011

Study Location: 1,034 clinical sites in 39 countries in North America, Latin America, Europe, and the Asian Pacific.

Who Was Studied: Patients with atrial fibrillation or flutter, plus at least one of the following additional risk factors for stroke: age of at least 75 years; previous stroke, transient ischemic attack, or systemic embolism; symptomatic heart failure within the previous 3 months or left ventricular ejection fraction of no more than 40%; diabetes mellitus; or hypertension requiring pharmacological treatment.

Who Was Excluded: Patients with atrial fibrillation due to a reversible cause, moderate or severe mitral stenosis, conditions other than atrial fibrillation that required anticoagulation (e.g., a prosthetic heart valve), stroke within the previous 7 days, requirement for aspirin at a dose of greater than 165 mg/day or for both aspirin and clopidogrel, or severe renal insufficiency.

How Many Patients: 18,201

Study Overview: See Figure 49.1 for a summary of the study design.

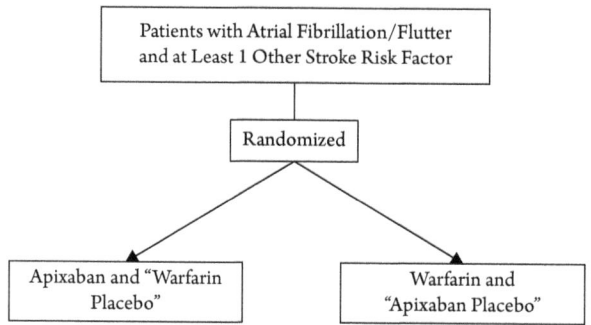

Figure 49.1 Summary of ARISTOTLE's Design.

Study Intervention: Patients in the apixaban group were administered apixaban and placebo; apixaban was given twice daily in 5 mg doses. A subset of patients received 2.5 mg doses if they fulfilled 2 or more of the following criteria: age at least 80 years, body weight ≤60 kg, or serum creatinine level of 1.5 mg/dL (133 μmol/L) or more. In addition to placebo, patients in the warfarin group were administered warfarin to achieve an INR of 2.0–3.0. INRs were monitored with the use of a blinded, encrypted, point-of-care INR device. The time that patients' INRs were within the therapeutic range was calculated by the Rosendaal method.[2] A program was implemented to improve the quality of INR control through education and feedback at site and country levels.

Follow-Up: Median of 1.8 years.

Endpoints: Primary efficacy outcome: ischemic or hemorrhagic stroke or systemic embolism. Secondary efficacy outcome: death from any cause. Primary safety outcome: major bleeding (defined according to the International Society on Thrombosis and Haemostasis [ISTH] criteria[3] as clinically overt bleeding accompanied by a decrease in the hemoglobin level of at least 2 g/dL or transfusion of at least 2 units of packed red cells, occurring at a critical site, or resulting in death). Secondary safety outcome: a composite of major bleeding and clinically relevant nonmajor bleeding (clinically overt bleeding that did not satisfy the criteria for major bleeding and that led to hospital admission, physician-guided medical or surgical treatment, or a change in antithrombotic therapy).

RESULTS

- The mean $CHADS_2$ score for study participants was 2.1. The $CHADS_2$ score, ranging from 1–6, predicts the risk of stroke in patients with atrial fibrillation, with higher scores indicating greater risk.[4]
- The rate of hemorrhagic stroke was 49% lower and the rate of ischemic or uncertain type of stroke was 8% lower in the apixaban group than in the warfarin group (although this did not reach statistical significance) (see Table 49.1).
- Fatal stroke occurred in 42 patients in the apixaban group and 67 patients in the warfarin group.
- The rate of intracranial hemorrhage was 0.33%/year in the apixaban group and 0.80% per year in the warfarin group (hazard ratio, 0.42; $P < 0.001$).
- The rate of any bleeding was 18.1% in the apixaban group and 25.8% in the warfarin group, an absolute reduction of 7.7% ($P < 0.001$).

Table 49.1. SUMMARY OF ARISTOTLE's KEY FINDINGS

Outcome	Event Rate by Group (%/Year)		Hazard Ratio	P Value
	Apixaban	Warfarin		
Primary efficacy outcome: stroke or systemic embolism	1.27%	1.60%	0.79	0.01
Secondary efficacy outcome: death from any cause	3.52%	3.94%	0.89	0.047
Primary safety outcome: ISTH[a] major bleeding	2.13%	3.09%	0.69	<0.001
Composite of stroke, systemic embolism, major bleeding, or death from any cause	6.13%	7.20%	0.85	<0.001

[a] International Society on Thrombosis and Haemostasis.

Criticisms and Limitations: Patients in the warfarin group had an INR in the therapeutic range (2.0–3.0) for a median of 66.0% of the time and a mean of 62.2% of the time. While this may seem low, it is similar to that of other studies involving warfarin.

Other Relevant Studies and Information:

- The key findings in ARISTOTLE are supported by a previous trial, AVERROES,[5] in which the same apixaban regimen, as compared with low-dose aspirin, was shown to significantly reduce the risk of stroke without any difference in the rates of major bleeding among high-risk patients with atrial fibrillation who were not warfarin candidates.
- As outlined in Chapter 48, in the RE-LY trial,[6] the oral direct thrombin inhibitor, dabigatran, was compared with warfarin. The twice-daily 150-mg dose of dabigatran reduced the rate of stroke but was associated with a similar overall rate of bleeding. The twice-daily 110-mg dose of dabigatran was associated with a similar rate of stroke but caused significantly less major bleeding than warfarin.
- As outlined in Chapter 50, in the ROCKET AF trial,[7] another oral factor Xa inhibitor, rivaroxaban, was compared to warfarin. Once-daily rivaroxaban was noninferior to warfarin in the prevention of stroke systemic embolism. The rates of intracranial hemorrhage and fatal bleeding were lower with rivaroxaban, but there was no advantage with respect to other major bleeding. The patients in the ROCKET AF study had, on average, more risk factors for stroke, with a mean $CHADS_2$ score of 3.5, versus 2.1 in the ARISTOTLE study.
- Apixaban is approved by the FDA for the prevention of stroke and systemic embolism in nonvalvular atrial fibrillation (NVAF), for the treatment of deep venous thrombosis (DVT) and pulmonary embolism (PE), and for prophylaxis against postoperative DVT/PE.
- Apixaban is endorsed as suitable first-line therapy for the prevention of stroke in NVAF in guidelines published by the American Academy of Neurology[8] and the American College of Cardiology/American Heart Association.[9]

Summary and Implications: In patients with atrial fibrillation and at least one other risk factor for stroke, apixaban significantly reduced the risk of stroke or systemic embolism by 21%, major bleeding by 31%, and death by 11% compared to warfarin.

CLINICAL CASE: STROKE PREVENTION IN ATRIAL FIBRILLATION

Case History:

A generally healthy 65-year-old man with a medical history of only well treated hypertension and noninsulin-dependent diabetes presented to his primary care doctor with 1 week of an intermittent fluttering sensation in his chest. He scheduled an urgent appointment with his primary care doctor, and electrocardiogram demonstrated atrial fibrillation.

Based on the results of this trial, what treatment options would you consider for this patient?

Suggested Answer:

This patient very likely will require anticoagulation. Apixaban should be strongly considered in place of warfarin based on the results of the ARISTOTLE study. This patient has a $CHADS_2$ score of 2 (for hypertension and diabetes), which closely mirrors the mean $CHADS_2$ score of 2.1 in ARISTOTLE. Furthermore, his otherwise benign medical history does not include any of the exclusionary conditions for apixaban in ARISTOTLE (such as mitral stenosis, a prosthetic valve, a need for high-dose aspirin, a recent stroke, or severe renal insufficiency). Based on the findings in ARISTOTLE, this patient would reduce his risk of stroke or systemic embolism, bleeding, and death by taking apixaban instead of warfarin.

References

1. Granger CB, Alexander JH, McMurray JJV, et al. Apixaban versus warfarin in patients with atrial fibrillation. *N Engl J Med*. 2011;365(11):981–992.
2. Rosendaal FR, Cannegieter SC, van der Meer FJ, Briët E. A method to determine the optimal intensity of oral anticoagulant therapy. *Thromb Haemost*. 1993;69(3): 236–239.
3. Schulman S, Kearon C; Subcommittee on Control of Anticoagulation of the Scientific and Standardization Committee of the International Society on Thrombosis and Haemostasis. Definition of major bleeding in clinical investigations of antihemostatic medicinal products in non-surgical patients. *J Thromb Haemost*. 2005;3(4):692–694.
4. Gage BF, van Walraven C, Pearce L, et al. Selecting patients with atrial fibrillation for anticoagulation: stroke risk stratification in patients taking aspirin. *Circulation*. 2004:110(16):2287-2292.
5. Connolly SJ, Eikelboom J, Joyner C, et al. Apixaban in patients with atrial fibrillation. *N Engl J Med*. 2011;364(9):806–817.

6. Connolly SJ, Ezekowitz MD, Yusuf S, et al. Dabigatran versus warfarin in patients with atrial fibrillation. *N Engl J Med.* 2009;361(12):1139–1151.
7. Patel MR, Mahaffey KW, Garg J, et al. Rivaroxaban versus warfarin in nonvalvular atrial fibrillation. *N Engl J Med.* 2011;365(10):883–891.
8. Culebras A, Messé SR, Chaturvedi S, Kase CS, Gronseth G. Summary of evidence-based guideline update: prevention of stroke in nonvalvular atrial fibrillation: report of the Guideline Development Subcommittee of the American Academy of Neurology. *Neurology.* 2014;82:716–724.
9. January CT, Wann LS, Alpert JS, et al. 2014 AHA/ACC/HRS guideline for the management of patients with atrial fibrillation: a report of the American College of Cardiology/American Heart Association Task Force on practice guidelines and the Heart Rhythm Society. *Circulation.* 2014. 130(23);e199–e267.

Rivaroxaban for Stroke Prevention in Atrial Fibrillation Patients
The ROCKET AF Trial
DANIEL C. BROOKS

> In patients with atrial fibrillation, rivaroxaban was noninferior to warfarin for the prevention of stroke or systemic embolism. There was no significant difference... in the risk of major bleeding, although intracranial and fatal bleeding occurred less frequently in the rivaroxaban group.
> —PATEL ET AL.[1]

Research Question: Is the oral factor Xa inhibitor rivaroxaban noninferior to warfarin in patients with nonvalvular atrial fibrillation in preventing ischemic or hemorrhagic stroke or systemic embolism?[1]

Funding: Johnson & Johnson Pharmaceutical Research and Bayer HealthCare.

Year Study Began: 2006

Year Study Published: 2011

Study Location: 1,178 participating sites in 45 countries

Who Was Studied: Patients with nonvalvular atrial fibrillation who were at moderate-to-high risk for stroke signified by a $CHADS_2$ score ≥2 (as mentioned in Chapter 49, the $CHADS_2$ score is a scale ranging from 1–6 in patients with atrial fibrillation with higher scores indicating a greater risk of embolic stroke).[2]

Who Was Excluded: Key exclusionary criteria included hemodynamically significant mitral stenosis, a prosthetic heart valve, atrial fibrillation due to a reversible cause, any stroke within 14 days, or transient ischemic attack within 3 days of randomization; indication for anticoagulation other than atrial fibrillation (e.g., venous thromboembolism); or requirement for an aspirin dose >100 mg/day.

How Many Patients: 14,264

Study Overview: See Figure 50.1 for a summary of the study design.

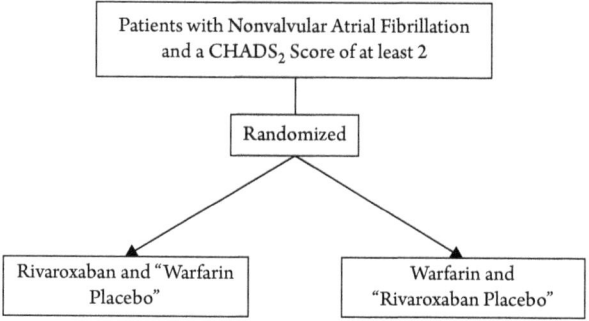

Figure 50.1 Summary of ROCKET AF's Design.

Study Intervention: Patients in the rivaroxaban group were administered fixed-dose rivaroxaban (20 mg/day or 15 mg/day in patients with a creatinine clearance of 30–49 mL/minute). Patients in the warfarin group received adjusted-dose warfarin to achieve a target INR of 2.0–3.0. Patients in each group also received a corresponding placebo to maintain blinding. All INR values for patients were tested with a device that sent the data to a central study monitor, who in turn provided study sites with real INRs for patients in the warfarin group and "sham INRs" for patients in the rivaroxaban group for medication "titration."

Follow-Up: Median of 707 days

Endpoints: Primary efficacy endpoint: a composite of stroke (ischemic or hemorrhagic) and systemic embolism. Secondary efficacy endpoints: a composite of stroke, systemic embolism, or death from cardiovascular causes; a composite of stroke, systemic embolism, death from cardiovascular causes, or myocardial infarction; and individual components of the composite endpoints. Primary safety endpoint: a composite of major and nonmajor clinically relevant bleeding events.

RESULTS

- The mean $CHADS_2$ score for study participants was 3.5.
- Rivaroxaban was not inferior to warfarin in achieving the primary endpoint of preventing stroke or systemic embolism. (see Table 50.1).
- Major bleeding from a gastrointestinal site was significantly more common in the rivaroxaban group versus the warfarin group (3.2% vs. 2.2%; $P <0.001$).
- Intracranial bleeding, however, was significantly lower in patients who received rivaroxaban vs. warfarin (0.5% vs 0.7%, $P=0.02$).
- There were increased rates of stroke or systemic embolism within 1 month of transition off of rivaroxaban compared with warfarin ($P=0.008$).

Table 50.1. SUMMARY OF ROCKET AF's KEY FINDINGS

Outcome	Group and Event Rate No./100 Patients		Hazard Ratio	P Value
	Rivaroxaban	Warfarin		
Primary efficacy endpoint: stroke or systemic embolism	1.7%	2.2%	0.79	<0.001 (noninferiority)
Primary safety endpoint: major and nonmajor clinically relevant bleeding	14.9%	14.5%	1.03	0.44
Any major bleeding	3.6%	3.4%	1.04	0.58
Intracranial hemorrhage	0.5%	0.7%	0.67	0.02
Fatal bleeding	0.2%	0.5%	0.50	0.003

Criticisms and Limitations: Patients in the warfarin group had an INR in the therapeutic range (2.0–3.0) for a median of 58% and a mean of 55% of the time. This was lower than the trial described in Chapter 49, ARISTOTLE,[3] which compared a different oral factor Xa inhibitor, apixiban, against warfarin.

Other Relevant Studies and Information:

- As outlined in Chapter 48, the RE-LY trial[4] compared the oral direct thrombin inhibitor, dabigatran, against warfarin. The twice-daily 150-mg dose of dabigatran reduced the rate of stroke but was associated with a similar overall rate of bleeding. The twice-daily 110-mg dose of dabigatran was associated with a similar rate of stroke and caused less major bleeding than warfarin. Dabigatran is the only noval oral anticoagulant that has decreased the risk of stroke to a statistically significant degree compared with warfarin.
- As outlined in Chapter 49, in the ARISTOTLE trial,[3] another oral factor Xa inhibitor, apixaban, was compared to warfarin. Twice-daily apixaban was found to be superior to warfarin in preventing stroke or systemic embolism, caused less bleeding, and resulted in less mortality. This was in the setting of patients being therapeutic on warfarin (INR between 2.0–3.0) for a greater average amount of time than in the ROCKET AF trial. However, the patients in the ROCKET AF study had, on average, more risk factors for stroke then the patients in the ARISTOTLE trial, with a mean $CHADS_2$ score of 3.5 in ROCKET AF versus 2.1 in the ARISTOTLE study.
- Rivaroxaban is approved by the FDA for the prevention of stroke and systemic embolism in nonvalvular atrial fibrillation (NVAF), for the treatment of deep venous thrombosis (DVT) and pulmonary embolism (PE), for the secondary prevention of DVT/PE, and for prophylaxis against postoperative DVT/PE.
- Rivaroxaban is an acceptable choice as first-line therapy for the prevention of stroke in NVAF in guidelines published by the American Academy of Neurology[5] and the American College of Cardiology/American Heart Association.[6]

Summary and Implications: In patients with nonvalvular atrial fibrillation who were at moderate-to-high risk for stroke, rivaroxaban was noninferior to warfarin in the prevention of ischemic or hemorrhagic stroke or systemic embolism. Rivaroxaban was associated with less intracranial hemorrhage than warfarin, but overall rates of major bleeding were similar.

CLINICAL CASE: STROKE PREVENTION IN ATRIAL FIBRILLATION

Case History:
A 76-year-old man with atrial fibrillation and a medical history of hypertension and a previous hospitalization for heart failure wanted to discuss options for anticoagulation other than warfarin. Several acquaintances of his were prescribed warfarin, and he did not want to undergo frequent INR monitoring or be too careful about his choices of food.

Based on the results of this trial, what treatment options would you consider for this patient?

Suggested Answer:
Anticoagulation is indicated for this patient as he is at moderate to high risk for stroke. His CHADS2 score is 3, which is near the mean $CHADS_2$ score in ROCKET AF. Rivaroxaban is an appropriate choice. As ROCKET AF demonstrated, rivaroxaban would be a noninferior choice compared to warfarin in decreasing his risk of stroke, and is overall associated with a similar risk of major bleeding. Rivaroxaban has an advantage over other novel oral anticoagulants in that it is taken only once daily.

References

1. Patel MR, Mahaffey KW, Garg J, et al. Rivaroxaban versus warfarin in nonvalvular atrial fibrillation. *N Engl J Med.* 2011;365(10):883–891.
2. Gage BF, van Walraven C, Pearce L, et al. Selecting patients with atrial fibrillation for anticoagulation: stroke risk stratification in patients taking aspirin. Circulation. 2004:110(16):2287-2292.
3. Granger CB, Alexander JH, McMurray JJV, et al. Apixaban versus warfarin in patients with atrial fibrillation. *N Engl J Med.* 2011;365(11):981–992.
4. Connolly SJ, Ezekowitz MD, Yusuf S, et al. Dabigatran versus warfarin in patients with atrial fibrillation. *N Engl J Med.* 2009;361(12):1139–1151.
5. Culebras A, Messé SR, Chaturvedi S, Kase CS, Gronseth G. Summary of evidence-based guideline update: prevention of stroke in nonvalvular atrial fibrillation: report of the Guideline Development Subcommittee of the American Academy of Neurology. *Neurology.* 2014;82:716–724.
6. January CT, Wann LS, Alpert JS, et al. 2014 AHA/ACC/HRS guideline for the management of patients with atrial fibrillation: a report of the American College of Cardiology/American Heart Association Task Force on practice guidelines and the Heart Rhythm Society. *Circulation.* 2014. 130(23);e199–e267.

Index

References to notes, tables, figures and boxes are denoted by an italicized *n, t, f,* and *b*

abortive therapy, acute migraine, 41, 45
ACAS trial (Asymptomatic Carotid Atherosclerosis Study), 289–94
ACTIVE W trial, 320, 321*n*2
acute bacterial meningitis, steroids for, 55–60
acute ischemic stroke
  aspirin *vs.* heparin for, 299–303
  case studies, 245, 250, 275, 298, 303, 315
  early aspirin for, 295–98
  endovascular therapy (Part I), 253–57
  endovascular therapy (Part II), 259–63
  endovascular therapy (Part III), 265–69
  endovascular therapy (Part IV), 271–76
  IMS III trial, 259–63
  IV thrombolysis 3–4.5 hours after, 247–51
  IV thrombolysis 3 hours after, 241–46
  lipid-lowering therapy, 315
  MR CLEAN trial, 271–76
  MR RESCUE trial, 265–69
  PROACT II trial, 253–57
acute optic neuritis, steroids for, 185–89
acute spinal cord injury, steroids *vs.* no steroids, 233–38
acyclovir, Bell's palsy, 49–53, 54*n*1, 54*n*8
AD Cooperative Study-Activities of Daily Living Inventory (ADCS-ADL), 14, 15*t*

AFFIRM trial, 102
alkylating chemotherapy, 177, 180–81
alteplase, intravenous, 244, 246*n*5, 247–50, 251*n*1, 251*n*6–7, 272
Alzheimer's disease
  case studies, 8, 16
  cholinesterase inhibitors in, 3–7
  diagnosis of, 17*n*2
  memantine for, 11–16
Alzheimer's Disease Assessment Scale (ADAS-Cog), 5–6, 7, 9*n*3
American Academy of Neurology, 18*n*16
  amyotrophic lateral sclerosis (ALS), 165, 167*n*5
  Bell palsy, 54*n*4
  dementia management, 18*n*16
  Guillain-Barré syndrome, 154, 156*n*6
  multiple sclerosis, 89, 91*n*8, 96, 98*n*6
  Parkinson's disease, 67, 75
  relapsing multiple sclerosis, 102, 104*n*6
  stroke prevention, 320, 321*n*6, 327, 328*n*4, 332, 334*n*8, 338, 339*n*5
American Association of Neurological Surgeons (AANS), 175, 233, 236, 293–94*n*5
American College of Cardiology, 293*n*5, 320, 321*n*7, 332, 334*n*9, 338, 339*n*6
American Headache Society, 44, 45*n*4

American Heart Association, 257n10, 280, 281n4, 286, 287n4, 293n5, 308, 310n11, 320, 321n7, 332, 334n9, 338, 339n6
American Stroke Association, 257n10, 280, 281n4, 286, 287n4, 293n5, 297, 302, 308, 310n11
Amin, Hardik P., 241–46, 277–81, 283–87
ampicillin, 56, 60n3
amyotrophic lateral sclerosis (ALS), riluzole for, 163–67
anterior cerebral circulation, 271–72
apixaban, 320
　stroke prevention in atrial fibrillation patients, 329–34
　warfarin vs., 329–32, 333n1, 339n3
Arch, Allison, 41–45, 253–57
ARISTOTLE trial, 329–34, 338
ASPECTS (Alberta Stroke Program Early CT Score), 262, 263n3
aspirin
　acute ischemic stroke, 295–98
　acute ischemic stroke, heparin vs., 299–303
　carotid stenosis, 284, 286, 290–91
　stroke prevention, 305–10
astrocytoma
　anaplastic, 180, 181n5
　WHO grade IV (glioblastoma), 172, 175, 178
ATLANTIS study (Alteplase Trombolysis for Acute Noninterventional Therapy in Ischemic Stroke), 246n5, 251n7–8
atorvastatin, after stroke or TIA, 311–15
atrial fibrillation patients
　apixaban for stroke prevention, 329–34
　dabigatran for stroke prevention, 323–28
　nonvalvular, 321n4, 321n6, 324, 327, 328, 328n4, 332, 338, 339n1, 339n5
　rivaroxaban for stroke prevention, 335–39
　warfarin for stroke prevention, 317–21
Australian trial, 127, 129–34
AVERROES, 332

bacterial meningitis, steroids for acute, 55–60
Bailey, Mary A., 105–9, 111–14, 115–19, 185–89
barbiturates, 22
Barthel Index, 243, 244t, 248, 273, 274t
Behavioral Rating Scale for Geriatric Patients (BGP), 14
Bell's palsy, steroids for, 49–54
benign paroxysmal positional vertigo (BPPV), Epley maneuver for, 193–99
benzodiazepines, 22, 213
bevacizumab, 174
BG-12 (dimethyl fumarate)
　relapsing-remitting MS (RRMS) treatment vs. placebo, 111–14
　RRMS treatment vs. placebo and glatiramer acetate, 115–19
Biomedicine and Health Programme (BIOMED 2), 123
Blond, Benjamin N, 49–54, 193–99
BPPV. See benign paroxysmal positional vertigo (BPPV)
brain cancer. See glioblastoma
Brain Trauma Foundation, 136, 138
BRANT trial (British Aneurysm Nimodipine), 145, 147n4
Brooks, Daniel C., 289–94, 317–21, 329–34, 335–39
Buckingham, Sarah E., 63–69, 71–77
bulbar-onset disease, 164–66

cabergoline, 67
Canalith Repositioning Procedure (CRP), 193–94, 195f, 196–98
CAPRIE study, 308, 310n10
carbamazepine, 27–31, 28f, 31n1, 31n10, 31n3–4, 31n6–7
carbidopa-levodopa, 64, 68, 69n11, 69n5, 76
cardiac arrest
　Australian trial, 129–34
　case study, 133
　HACA trial, 123–28
　hypothermia protocol, 125f, 130f, 132

INDEX

neurologic outcome after, 123, 125–27, 128n1, 129, 131–32
normothermia protocol, 123, 125–27, 130–32
therapeutic hypothermia for, 123–28, 129–34
carotid endarterectomy
 for asymptomatic carotid stenosis, 289–94
 for symptomatic high-grade carotid stenosis, 277–81
 for symptomatic moderate carotid stenosis, 283–87
carotid stenosis
 carotid endarterectomy for asymptomatic, 289–94
 carotid endarterectomy for high-grade, 277–81
 carotid endarterectomy for moderate, 283–87
 case study, 286
case studies
 abortive therapy for migraine headache, 45
 acute ischemic stroke, aspirin vs. heparin, 303
 acute ischemic stroke, aspirin vs. placebo, 298
 acute ischemic stroke, endovascular therapy for, 275
 acute ischemic stroke, IV thrombolysis 3–4.5 hours after, 250
 acute ischemic stroke, IV thrombolysis 3 hours after, 245
 acute ischemic stroke, lipid-lowering therapy after, 315
 apixaban for stroke prevention in atrial fibrillation, 333
 asymptomatic carotid stenosis, 293
 Bell's palsy treatment, 53–54
 benign paroxysmal positional vertigo (BPPV) treatment, 198
 carotid endarterectomy for symptomatic carotid stenosis, 286
 cholinesterase inhibitors in Alzheimer's disease, 8

clinically isolated demyelinating event, 90
clinically isolated syndrome, 97
continuous dopamine agonist for restless legs syndrome, 214
dabigatran for stroke prevention in atrial fibrillation, 328
decompressive craniectomy for diffuse TBI, 139
dexamethasone for acute bacterial meningitis, 59
glioblastoma, chemotherapy for, 175
glioblastoma, methylated *MGMT* gene promoter and temozolomide in, 181
Guillain-Barré syndrome, 155
initial treatment of newly diagnosed partial epilepsy, 30–31
memantine for Alzheimer's disease, 16
modafinil for narcolepsy, 206
multiple sclerosis, fingolimod for relapsing, 108
multiple sclerosis, methylprednisolone for relapses of, 85
multiple sclerosis, oral BG-12 for relapsing, 118
multiple sclerosis (relapsing-remitting) and natalizumab, 103
myasthenia gravis, 160
nimodipine for subarachnoid hemorrhage, 146
Parkinson's disease, levodopa for recently diagnosed, 68
Parkinson's disease, management of advanced, 76
riluzole in ALS, 166
rivaroxaban for stroke prevention in atrial fibrillation, 339
sciatica patient, 223
steroids for acute optic neuritis, 188
stroke prevention, aspirin and dipyridamole, 309
surgery for lumbar degenerative spondylolisthesis, 231
therapeutic hypothermia for post-cardiac arrest, 133

case studies (*Cont.*)
  treatment of overt generalized status epilepticus, 24
  valproate therapy for epilepsy, 36
  warfarin for stroke prevention in atrial fibrillation, 320
CAST trial (Chinese Acute Stroke Trial), 295–98, 301–2, 303n2
Cerebral Performance Categories (CPC) Scale, 125t, 126
cerebrospinal fluid (CSF), 155, 227
CHADS score, 320, 331–33, 336–39
CHAMPS Trial, 87–91
Chan, Amy, 27–31, 171–76
CHANCE trial, 297
chemotherapy, glioblastoma, 174, 175, 176n4, 177–81, 181n4–5
cholinesterase inhibitors, Alzheimer's disease, 3–8
cilengitide, 175
Claycomb, Robert J., 55–60, 99–104, 305–10, 323–28
Clinical Dementia Rating scale Sum of Boxes (CDR-SB), 5–6
Clinical Global Impressions (CGI), 210–12, 215n3
clinically definite multiple sclerosis (CDMS), 88–90, 93–97
clinically isolated syndrome (CIS), glatiramer acetate for, 93–98
Clinician's Interview-Based Impression of Change Plus Caregiver Input (CIBIC-Plus), 5–7, 14
clonazepam, 30, 213
clopidogrel, 297, 298n5, 308–9, 310n9–10, 320, 321n2, 330
CONFIRM trial, 115–19
Congress of Neurological Surgeons (CNS), 175, 233, 236, 293–94n5
continuous dopamine agonist, restless legs syndrome (RLS), 209–15
corticosteroids
  acute optic neuritis, 85n4
  bacterial meningitis, 55–56, 58, 59, 60n3, 60n6
  Bell's palsy, 53
  clinically isolated syndrome, 97
  Guillain-Barré syndrome, 152
  multiple sclerosis, 103
  optic neuritis, 185, 187–88, 189n1
craniectomy, decompressive, for traumatic brain injury, 135–39
CRP. *See* Canalith Repositioning Procedure (CRP)
cyclosporine, 161n2

dabigatran, 320, 321n3, 332, 334n6, 338, 339n4
  stroke prevention in atrial fibrillation patients, 323–28
  warfarin *vs.*, 323–25, 326t, 327, 328n1, 334n4, 339n4
daytime sleepiness, 203, 207n1, 207n4
decompressive craniectomy, traumatic brain injury (TBI), 135–39
DECRA trial, 135–39
deep-brain stimulation, for Parkinson's disease, 71–77
deep venous thrombosis (DVT), 307, 332, 338
DEFINE trial, 111–14, 117–18, 119n5–6
DEFUSE 2 study, 268, 269n6
demyelinating event, interferon beta-1a for, 87–91
dexamethasone, acute bacterial meningitis, 55–59, 56f, 57t, 58t, 59n1, 60n5
diazepam, status epilepticus, 21, 22f, 23t, 24
dimethyl fumarate. *See* BG-12 (dimethyl fumarate)
dipyridamole, stroke prevention, 305–10
disk herniation, 219, 224n3–4
Dix-Hallpike maneuver, 194, 197, 198
donepezil, Alzheimer's disease, 3, 4f, 5–8, 9n1, 9n5, 9n7, 11–12, 14f, 16, 17n1, 18n16–18
dopaminergic agonists, 209, 213–14
Down's syndrome, 15, 18n15
DSM-III-R (*Diagnostic and Statistical Manual of Mental Disorders*, 3rd ed. revised), 3, 4
Dyskinesia Scale, 73, 74t

INDEX

Eastern Cooperative Oncology Group (ECOG), 178, 181*n*3
ECASS III trial, 244, 247–51
EDS. *See* excessive daytime sleepiness (EDS)
electroencephalogram (EEG), generalized status epilepticus, 22, 23
endovascular therapy for acute ischemic stroke
  case study, 275
  part I (intra-arterial thrombolysis), 253–57
  part II (after IV thrombolysis), 259–63
  part III (using neuroimaging for patient selection), 265–69
  part IV (clinical trial success), 271–76
enzastaurin, 174
epilepsy
  case studies, 30–31, 36
  lamotrigine for partial, 27–31
  valproate for, 33–37
Epley maneuver
  benign paroxysmal positional vertigo (BPPV), 193–99
  diagram of canalith repositioning procedure, 195*f*
Epworth Sleepiness Scale (ESS), 204, 205*t*, 207*n*4
erlotinib, 175
ESPRIT study, 308, 310*n*7–8
ESPS-2 trial (European Stroke Prevention Study), 305–10
ESS. *See* Epworth Sleepiness Scale (ESS)
European Carotid Surgery Trial (ECST), 280, 281*n*3, 285, 286, 287*n*3
European Federation of Neurological Societies, 154, 156*n*7
EuroQol Group 5-Dimension Self-Report Questionnaire, 273, 274*t*
everolimus, 175
excessive daytime sleepiness (EDS), 203–4, 206
Expanded Disability Status Scale (EDSS)
  multiple sclerosis, 82–84, 95, 100–101, 103, 105–6, 109*n*2
  relapsing-remitting multiple sclerosis, 112, 115

facial nerve grading system, House-Brackmann, 51*t*
Farooque, Pue, 21–25
fingolimod, relapsing multiple sclerosis, 105–9
frontotemporal lobar degeneration (FTLD), 15

gabapentin, 28*f*, 29, 31*n*1, 213
gadolinium, MRI with, 85, 88, 94, 97, 181
gadolinium-enhancing lesion, 88, 89*t*, 95, 101*t*, 103, 108, 112, 116
gebitinib, 174
generalized status epilepticus, lorazepam for, 21–24
German Society of Neurology, 72, 75
Ghoshal, Shivani, 33–37, 135–39
Glasgow Coma Scale (GCS), 136
Glasgow Outcome Scale, 56, 57*t*, 135–36, 243, 244*t*, 248
Glasgow Outcome Scale - Extended (GOSE), 135, 136, 137*t*, 138*t*
glatiramer acetate
  BG-12 *vs.*, in RRMS, 115–18, 119*n*1, 119*n*5
  clinically definite multiple sclerosis (CDMS), 91*n*7
  for clinically isolated syndrome, 89, 93–98
glioblastoma
  case studies, 175, 181
  methylated *MGMT* gene promoter and temozolomide in, 177–81
  radiotherapy plus temozolomide, 171–76
  WHO grade IV astrocytoma, 172, 175, 178
Grant, Ryan A., 225–32
Guillain-Barré syndrome, intravenous immunoglobulin (IVIG) *vs.* plasma exchange, 151–56

HACA trial (Hypothermia after Cardiac Arrest), 123–28, 132, 133
Hachinski Ischemia Score, 13*t*
Hani, Abeer J., 203–7

headache, sumatriptan for acute
    migraine, 41–45
hemorrhage, nimodipine for
    subarachnoid, 141–47
heparin, 242, 248
    acute ischemic stroke, 253–56, 298n2,
        299–303
Hochman, Michael E., 247–51
Hoehn and Yahr Scale, 63–64, 64f, 68n2
House-Brackmann Facial Nerve Grading
    System, 50, 51t, 52t
Hwang, David Y., 253–57, 259–63,
    265–69, 271–76
hydantoin, 22
hypothermia. *See* therapeutic
    hypothermia for cardiac arrest
Hypothermia after Cardiac Arrest. *See*
    HACA trial

IMS (Interventional Management
    of Stroke)–III trial, 259–63,
    268, 274–75
interferon beta-1a
    clinically definite multiple sclerosis
        (CDMS), 93, 96, 97
    demyelinating event, 87–91
    relapsing multiple sclerosis, 99–101,
        103, 104n1, 104n3, 105–8
interferon beta-1b, clinically definite
    multiple sclerosis (CDMS),
    93, 96, 97
International Headache Society, 41
International League Against Epilepsy
    (ILAE), 29, 31, 31n11, 31n5, 37n2
International Liaison Committee
    on Resuscitation, 127, 128n7,
    132, 134n7
International Restless Legs Syndrome
    Study Group (IRLSSG), 209–10,
    213, 215n2, 215n6
International Society on Thrombosis
    and Haemostasis (ISTH), 331,
    331t, 333n3
intra-arterial thrombolysis, acute ischemic
    stroke, 253–57
intracranial aneurysm, 141–42

intracranial hemorrhage, 242, 248, 249t,
    255–56, 266, 275, 300, 302, 319t,
    331–32, 337t, 338
intracranial pressure, 135–39
intravenous immunoglobulin (IVIG)
    Guillain-Barré syndrome, 151–56
    myasthenia gravis, 157–61
intravenous thrombolysis, endovascular
    therapy for acute ischemic
    stroke, 259–63
ipsilateral stroke, 279, 284–85,
    289, 291–93
IRLSSG. *See* International Restless Legs
    Syndrome Study Group (IRLSSG)
ischemic stroke. *See* acute ischemic stroke;
    endovascular therapy for acute
    ischemic stroke; stroke
IST trial (International Stroke Trial), 297,
    298n2, 299–303

Kalp, Matthew D., 259–63,
    265–69, 271–76
Kolb, Luis, 219–24
Kruskal-Wallis Test, 187t

lamotrigine, partial epilepsy, 27–31, 31n1,
    31n4, 31n9–10, 33, 34t, 35t
Landreneau, Mark, 295–98, 299–303
levetiracetam, 24, 29, 31n3, 31n6,
    35, 36
levodopa, 63–69, 213. *See also*
    carbidopa-levodopa
Lewy bodies, 15, 17–18n10
limb-onset disease, 164–66
lorazepam, 21–24
Lovinger, Joshua, 11–18, 81–85, 177–81
Low Back Pain Bothersome Scale, 227
lumbar degenerative spondylolisthesis,
    surgery for, 225–32
lumbar disc herniation, 224n2–6
lumbar spine, 229, 231n3,
    232n12–13, 232n6

Mac Grory, Brian, 163–67, 311–15
Maine Lumbar Spine Study, 229,
    232n12–13, 232n6

Maintenance of Wakefulness Test (MWT), 204–6
MASCIS II trial, 233–38
mechanical thrombectomy, 256, 257n5, 272
Medical Outcomes Study 36-Item Short-Form General Health Survey (SF-36), 220, 226–27, 228t, 231n2
memantine, Alzheimer's disease, 11, 14–16, 17n1, 17n4, 17n6–7, 17–18n10, 18n12, 18n15–18, 18n20–21
MERCI retriever, 260, 269n3–4, 276n2–3
methylated *MGMT* gene promoter, 174, 175, 176n3
  case study, 181
  temozolomide and, for glioblastoma, 177–81
methylprednisolone
  meningitis, 60n4
  multiple sclerosis, 82, 82f, 83t, 84, 85, 85n1, 85n3, 85n5, 88f, 90
  optic neuritis, 185–88
  spinal cord injury, 233–37, 237n2–3, 238n10, 238n4–8
MGMT (O^6-methylguanine-DNA methyltransferase) gene. *See* methylated *MGMT* gene promoter
middle cerebral artery, 248, 253–54, 256, 260, 262, 266, 275, 286, 328
migraine, sumatriptan for acute, 41–45
Mini-Mental State Examination (MMSE), 5–8, 12, 15–16, 18n17–18
modafinil, narcolepsy, 203–7
modified Hoehn and Yahr Scale, 63–64, 64f, 68n2
modified Rankin Scale (mRS), 243, 244t, 248, 249t, 254, 255t, 261, 267, 267t, 268, 273, 312
mortality
  acute ischemic stroke, 243–44, 248, 249t, 255t, 267, 273, 275, 296–97, 313–15
  amyotrophic lateral sclerosis, 164
  atrial fibrillation, 329, 338
  bacterial meningitis, 57t, 58
  cardiac arrest, 126t, 127, 132

  carotid stenosis, 280, 286, 289
  epilepsy, 23
  Guillain-Barré syndrome, 153
  spinal cord injury, 235
  traumatic brain injury, 136
MR CLEAN trial, 271–76
MR RESCUE trial, 265–69, 275
mRS. *See* modified Rankin Scale (mRS)
Multiple Sclerosis Council for Clinical Practice, 89, 91n8, 96
Multiple Sclerosis Functional Composite (MSFC), 106
multiple sclerosis (MS)
  case studies, 85, 90, 97, 103, 108, 118
  clinically definite multiple sclerosis (CDMS), 88–90, 93–97
  fingolimod for relapsing, 105–9
  glatiramer acetate for clinically isolated syndrome, 93–98
  interferon beta-1a for first demyelinating event, 87–91
  natalizumab for relapsing-remitting, 99–104
  oral *vs.* IV steroids for relapses of, 81–85
  See also relapsing-remitting multiple sclerosis (RRMS)
Mulukutla, Sarah A., 87–91, 93–98
myasthenia gravis, intravenous immunoglobulin (IVIG) *vs.* plasma exchange, 157–61

naloxone, 233–35, 237n2–3
narcolepsy, modafinil for, 203–7
NASCET trial (North American Symptomatic Carotid Endarterectomy Trial)
  design, 278f, 284f
  high-grade carotid stenosis, 277–81
  moderate carotid stenosis, 283–87
NASCIS II trial (National Acute Spinal Cord Injury Study), 233–38, 235t, 237n2–3, 238n6, 238n8
natalizumab, for relapsing multiple sclerosis, 99–104

National Institute of Neurological and Communicative Disorders and Stroke-Alzheimer's Disease and Related Disorders Association (NINCDS-ADRDA), 3–4, 12, 12b, 17n2
National Institute of Neurological Disorders and Stroke (NINDS). See NINDS trial
National Institutes of Health Stroke Scale (NIHSS), 242–43, 244t, 245, 248–49, 251n2, 254, 255t, 256, 260–62, 266, 272–73, 274t, 275
Neisseria meningitidis, 58t
neuroimaging, MR RESCUE trial, 265–69
neurologic outcome
   cardiac arrest, 123, 125–27, 128n1, 129, 131–32
   ischemic stroke, 241, 244t
   spinal cord injury, 235t
   subarachnoid hemorrhage, 143t, 144t
neurostimulation, Parkinson's disease, 71–76
nifedipine, 147n3
NIHSS. See National Institutes of Health Stroke Scale (NIHSS)
nimodipine, subarachnoid hemorrhage, 141–47
NINCDS-ADRDA (National Institute of Neurological and Communicative Disorders and Stroke-Alzheimer's Disease and Related Disorders Association), 3–4, 12, 12b, 17n2
NINDS (National Institute of Neurological Disorders and Stroke) trial, 17, 241–46, 249, 250, 251n8, 256
NOA-08 trial, 180, 181n5
nonvalvular atrial fibrillation, 321n4, 321n6, 324, 327–28, 328n4, 332, 338, 339n1, 339n5
Nordic trial, 180, 181n6
normothermia protocol, after cardiac arrest, 123, 125–27, 130–32

North American Spine Society (NASS), 230, 231n3, 232n15
North American Symptomatic Carotid Endarterectomy Trial. See NASCET Trial

O^6-methylguanine-DNA methyltransferase gene. See methylated *MGMT* gene promoter
Omay, Sacit Bulent, 233–38
ONTT trial (Optic Neuritis Treatment Trial), 84–85, 185, 186f, 187–88, 189n2
optic neuritis, 90, 185–89
Optic Neuritis Treatment Trial. See ONTT trial
Oswestry Disability Index (ODI), 227, 228t, 232n11
oxcarbazepine, 28f, 29, 31n1

Parkinson disease dementia, 17–18n10
parkinsonism, 17n9
Parkinson's disease
   case studies, 68, 76
   dementia, 15
   levodopa for, 63–69
Parkinson's Disease Questionnaire (PDQ-39), 73, 74t, 76n3
PD MED Collaborative Group, 67, 69n9
Penumbra System, 260, 266, 267t
phenobarbital, 21, 22f, 23t, 24, 30
phenytoin, 21, 22f, 23t, 24, 29
plasma exchange
   Guillain-Barré syndrome, 151–56
   myasthenia gravis, 157–61
plasmapheresis, 156n2, 161n5
Pneumocystis carinii, 173, 175
PPST (penumbra pivotal stroke trial), 257n4
pramipexole, 67, 68n3, 69n4, 213
PreCISe trial (patients with clinically isolated syndrome), 89, 91n7, 93–98, 97n1
prednisolone, Bell's palsy, 49–54, 54n1, 54n3, 54n5, 54n7

prednisone, 54n6, 83–84, 88f, 160, 185–88
pregabalin, 29, 31n9, 213
primidone, 30
PROACT II trial (Prolyse in Acute Cerebral Thromboembolism), 253–57
PRoFESS study, 308
progressive multifocal leukoencephalopathy (PML), 102t, 102–3, 104n7
prourokinase, 253, 257n1

Quantitative Myasthenia Gravis Score (QMGS), 157–59, 159t
radicular pain, 223
radiculopathy, 226–27, 230–31
radiotherapy, temozolomide and, for glioblastoma, 171–76

Ranpura, Ashish L., 3–9, 209–15
relapsing-remitting multiple sclerosis (RRMS)
  CONFIRM trial, 115–19
  DEFINE trial, 111–14
  fingolimod for, 105–9
  natalizumab for, 99–104
  oral BG-12 (dimethyl fumarate) for, 111–14, 115–19
  see also multiple sclerosis (MS)
RE-LY trial, 323–28, 332
RESCUE-ICP (Randomized Evaluation of Surgery with Craniectomy for Uncontrollable Elevation of Surgery with Craniectomy), 138, 139
restless legs syndrome (RLS)
  continuous dopamine agonist for, 209–15
  rotigotine for, 209, 211f, 211–14, 215n1
riluzole, amyotrophic lateral sclerosis (ALS), 163–67
rivaroxaban, 320
  stroke prevention in atrial fibrillation patients, 335–39
  warfarin *vs.*, 334n7, 335–39, 339n1

RLS. *See* restless legs syndrome (RLS)
Robeson, Kimberly R., 157–61
ROCKET AF trial, 320, 335–39
Roland Disability Questionnaire for Sciatica, 220, 221t
ropinirole, 67, 213, 214
rotigotine, restless legs syndrome, 209, 211f, 211–14, 215n1
RRMS. *See* relapsing-remitting multiple sclerosis (RRMS)

SANAD trial
  Arm A of, 27–31
  Arm B of, 33–36
Sandoglobulin (intravenous immunoglobulin), 152, 156n1
Schwab and England Scale, 73, 74t
sciatica
  conservative treatment, 219–23, 224n1, 224n6
  early surgery for, 219–24
scopolamine, 194
Semont maneuver, 197
SENTINEL trial, 99–104
Severe Impairment Battery (SIB), 14, 15t, 18n12
SF-36. *See* Medical Outcomes Study 36-Item Short-Form General Health Survey (SF-36)
simvastatin, 245
SPAF III (Stroke Prevention in Atrial Fibrillation) trial, 317–21
SPARCL (Stroke Prevention by Aggressive Reduction in Cholesterol Levels) trial, 311–15
spinal cord injury, steroids *vs.* no steroids for acute, 233–38
spine disorders
  early surgery for sciatica, 219–24
  steroids *vs.* no steroids for spinal cord injury, 233–38
  surgery for lumbar degenerative spondylolisthesis, 225–32
Spine Patient Outcomes Research Trial (SPORT), 224n3–4, 232n7, 232n9

spondylolisthesis, surgery for lumbar degenerative, 225–32
SPORT trial, 225–32
statins, 245, 279, 285, 309, 311–15
status epilepticus, lorazepam for generalized, 21–24
Stenosis Bothersomeness Index, 227
steroids
  for acute bacterial meningitis, 55–60
  for acute optic neuritis, 185–89
  for Bell's palsy, 49–54
  oval vs. IV for multiple sclerosis relapses, 81–85
Streptococcus pneumoniae, 57, 58t
stroke
  apixaban for prevention in atrial fibrillation patients, 329–34
  atorvastatin after, 311–15
  dabigatran for prevention in atrial fibrillation patients, 323–28
  dipyridamole and aspirin for prevention, 305–10
  ipsilateral, 279, 284–85, 289, 291–93
  rivaroxaban for prevention in atrial fibrillation patients, 335–39
  warfarin for prevention in atrial fibrillation patients, 317–21
  see also acute ischemic stroke; endovascular therapy for acute ischemic stroke
subarachnoid hemorrhage, nimodipine for, 141–47
subthalamic nucleus, 72, 75–76, 77n4–5
sumatriptan, acute migraine, 41–45
surgery
  lumbar degenerative spondylolisthesis, 225–32
  sciatica, 219–24
surgical decompression, 226, 229–30
Swedish Aspirin Low-Dose Trial (SALT), 310n6

T2-weighted hyperintense lesion, 8, 88, 89t, 94, 97, 113t, 117t
temozolomide

methylated *MGMT* gene promoter and, for glioblastoma, 177–81
  radiotherapy and, for glioblastoma, 171–76
temsirolimus, 175
therapeutic hypothermia for cardiac arrest
  Australian trial, 129–34
  HACA trial, 123–28
THRaST study (Thrombolysis and Statins), 314, 315n3
Thrombolysis in Cerebral Infarction (TICI), 261, 267, 274
TIA. *See* transient ischemic attack (TIA)
TIMI grade (Thrombolysis in Myocardial Infarction), 254, 255t
tissue plasminogen activator, 241, 245n1, 251n4–5, 256, 257n2, 257n8
topiramate, 28f, 29, 31n1, 33, 34t, 35t, 36, 37n1, 309
TRANSFORMS trial, 105–8
transient ischemic attack (TIA)
  apixaban, 330
  aspirin, 298n5, 305–6, 310n5, 318–19
  carotid endarterectomy, 277–78, 281n4, 284, 287n4, 291
  dabigatran, 324–25
  dipyridamole, 305–6
  high-dose atorvastatin after, 311–15
  rivaroxaban, 336
  warfarin, 318–19
traumatic brain injury (TBI)
  decompressive craniectomy for diffuse, 135–39
  Glasgow Outcome Scale - Extended (GOSE), 135, 136, 137t, 138t
TREVO 2, 269n3, 276n3

Unified Parkinson's Disease Rating Scale (UPDRS), 64–65, 66t, 67, 68
  (UPDRS–II), 73, 74t
  (UPDRS–III), 73, 74t
US Modafinil in Narcolepsy Multicenter Study Group, 206, 207n6–7

INDEX

valacyclovir, 52, 54n3, 54n5, 54n7
valproate, epilepsy, 28f, 33–37, 34t
ventricular fibrillation (VF), 123–24, 127, 130, 133
vertigo. *See* benign paroxysmal positional vertigo (BPPV)
Veterans Affairs Cooperative Study, 292, 293n2
vigabatrin, 30
visual analogue scale (VAS) for leg pain, 220, 221f, 222

warfarin
    apixaban *vs.*, 329–32, 333n1, 339n3
    dabigatran *vs.*, 323–25, 326t, 327, 328n1, 334n6, 339n4
    rivaroxaban *vs.*, 334n7, 335–39, 339n1
    stroke prevention in atrial fibrillation patients, 317–21
WHO grade IV astrocytoma (glioblastoma), 172, 175, 178
Willis-Ekbom disease, 215n6
World Health Organization Performance Status, cancer, 173t

Yang, Irene Hwa, 151–56
Youn, Teddy S., 123–28, 129–34, 141–47

zonisamide, 29, 31n7, 36

www.ingramcontent.com/pod-product-compliance
Ingram Content Group UK Ltd.
Pitfield, Milton Keynes, MK11 3LW, UK
UKHW021316180426
11947UKWH00015B/1268